HEAL
with
AMINO
ACIDS
and Nutrients

Survive Stress, Pain, Anxiety, Depression
Without Drugs
What to Use and When

Billie J. Sahley, Ph.D.
Katherine M. Birkner, C.R.N.A., Ph.D.

Pain & Stress Publications®
San Antonio, Texas
2000

Note to Readers

This material is not intended to replace services of a physician, nor is it meant to encourage diagnosis and treatment of illness, disease or other medical problems by the layman. This book should not be regarded as a substitute for professional medical treatment and while every care is taken to ensure the accuracy of the content, the authors and the publisher cannot accept legal responsibility for any problem arising out of experimentation with the methods described. Any application of the recommendations set forth in the following pages is at the reader's discretion and sole risk. If you are under a physician's care for any condition, he or she can advise you as to whether the programs described in this book are suitable for you.

This publication has been compiled through research resources at the **Pain & Stress Center**, San Antonio, Texas 78229.

5th Printing, June, 2000
Printed in U.S.A

A Pain & Stress Publication®
Vickie Worthington, Editor

Additional copies may be ordered from:
Pain & Stress Center
5282 Medical Drive, Suite 160, San Antonio, TX 78229-6023
1-800-669-2256 *OR*
visit Pain & Stress Center website: http://www.painstresscenter.com

Library of Congress Number 00-103714
ISBN 1-889391-19-0

Acknowledgments and Dedication

Many people pass through our lives whose influence leaves a positive imprint that we carry with us. We dedicate and acknowledge those gifted people for their support, guidance, and dedication to making this world a better place to live and raise our children.

The authors would like to express special thanks to the people who helped make this book possible:

To a new generation of physicians, therapists and educators who seek to find the natural alternative that frees the addicted from the prison of prescription drugs and gives them God's greatest gift—*the freedom to make a choice.*

To Robert Michael Benson, M.D. who taught me how to live my impossible dream.

To Julian Whitaker, M.D., one of God's gifted healers and an inspiration to all those who reach out.

To Candace Pert, Ph.D., neuroscientist, whose research opened many doors in amino acids and neuropeptides.

To David E. Bresler, Ph.D., our mentor in chronic pain and integral medicine.

To Doris J. Rapp, M.D., whose wisdom and teachings opened the door to the world of environmental medicine.

To Sherry Rogers, M.D. who introduced us to the world of magnesium chloride.

To Burton Goldberg, Ph.D., publisher and teacher, for his dedication to the fields of alternative medicine and healing.

Linda M. Volpenhein, C.N.C. whose tireless hours of assistance helped make this book a reality.

To a little boy named Scooter, now, an angel in heaven.

And to the Lord, for always lighting ours paths.

Table of Contents

Introduction

The late Carl Pfeiffer, M.D., Ph.D., known throughout the world for his work with amino acids and brain chemistry summarized *orthomolecular therapy* as a means of supplying the brain and cells with the right mixture of nutrients. Dr. Pfeiffer stated, "Many diseases are known to be the wrong balance of essential amino acids and nutrients in the body. Adjusting the diet, eliminating junk foods and ingesting the proper doses of essential vitamins, minerals and amino acids, can correct the chemical imbalance of disease."

The orthomolecular approach helps patients become more aware of our dangerously polluted environment and nutrient-stripped refined foods. The orthomolecular approach is both, corrective and preventative. Meganutrient therapy has become a part of orthomolecular medicine. While it is becoming widely recognized that orthomolecular therapy cures patients by correcting brain chemical imbalances, it is little known that in certain combinations meganutrients can be as immediately effective as potent painkillers or tranquilizers. Meganutrients treat the whole person's biochemical imbalances; they can be of immediate and long-term benefit. The type of treatment offered by orthomolecular doctors and therapists varies, but the mainstream of work focuses upon meganutrient therapy and diagnostic tests, and treatment with adequate nutrients is a distinguishing characteristic of orthomolecular medicine.

Orthomolecular therapy takes into consideration that every individual is biochemically unique. Every patient has a very different nutrient and amino acid requirement. With application of this therapy, each individual's need is met, and the mind and body are in a state of homeostasis—a condition where everything in the body is in balance and capable of resisting environmental changes, while regulating internal metabolic function.

In *Orthomolecular Medicine for Physicians* Dr. Hoffer states, "Every tissue of the body is affected by nutrition. Under conditions of poor nutrition, the kidneys stop filtering, the stomach stops digesting, the adrenals stop secreting, and other organs follow suit."

Good nutrition is essential to the preservation of health and the prevention of disease. Meganutrient therapy has become a part of orthomolecular medicine. It has continually expanded and now recognizes that all of our biological interactions with food, water, air, and light are an important part of good health and prevention of illness, if taken in proper amounts.

Special Information

The major focus of this book is amino acids and nutrients. As you will notice at times we discuss the use of herbs, vitamins, minerals and other important nutrients. We included this important information so that you would be aware of all available options for maximum benefit. All of the products described in this book are used at the Pain & Stress Center in our orthomolecular program.

One of the major functions of the Pain & Stress Center is research. Our goal through research is to supply our readers, patients and customers with the latest information to help you and your family achieve optimum health. *If you have any questions regarding any of the products discussed in this book,* call the Pain & Stress Center at 1-800-669-2256.

You will notice under some conditions such as Depression, we mention several products. *This does not mean you need all of the products. Use the nutrients that fit your symptoms.* You may find some work better for you than others. Everyone is biochemically unique, and responds to supplements in a different way. Our goal is to give you all of the information available to help you find the best and most effective resources for you.

Neurotransmitters, Brain Language

Amino acids and brain function go hand in hand. Understanding your brain function gives you a more comprehensive picture of how to use various amino acids to effectively treat pain, stress, anxiety, and depression. Your body needs and uses basic nutrients every day. These include vitamins, minerals, proteins, carbohydrates, and fats. If you were to take the water and fat out of your body, 75% of the remainder would be protein. Muscles, cell membranes, enzymes, and the neurotransmitters are all proteins.

The brain controls every cell in the human body. Its commanding presence is responsible for all sensation, movement, thought, behavior, and a lifetime of memories and dreams. The importance of a healthy, well-nourished, efficiently functioning brain cannot be overstated. This three-pound powerpack comprises less than 2% of your total body weight. Your brain regulates your breathing, heartbeat, body temperature and hormone balance. Speech at any level would be impossible without needed nutrients for proper brain function.

Yet, in spite of the absolute importance of a smoothly functioning brain, it is the most poorly nourished organ in the human body. Ten billion neurons (brain cells) cry to be fed constantly. They need amino acids, vitamins, minerals, oxygen, and fatty acids. The neurons' needs must be satisfied every minute of every day of your entire life. All these nutrients are supplied to the brain via the bloodstream. If blood-flow to the brain is interrupted even for 20 seconds, unconsciousness will result. If this mighty powerpack is deprived of blood or oxygen for more than 7 to 10 minutes, it will die. The brain feeds on energy in the form of the chemical ATP, adenosine triphosphate. This energy fuels the neurotransmitters, the chemical language of the brain, conducts electrical impulses, transports proteins throughout the cells, extends new nerve connections to other brain cells, and rebuilds worn-out cell membranes. The brain must create its own energy for the billions of neurons that it must feed, and cannot borrow or steal this energy from other parts of the body.

How does the brain make this energy? Inside each neuron resides hundreds of little structures called *mitochondria*. These function as power plants for the cells. These little power plants burn fuel to generate the crucial ATP energy. The brain's very life depends on it. While virtually all organs and tissues of the human body can burn either fat or sugar for fuel, the brain can burn only sugar (glucose) under normal, nonfasting conditions. This glucose requirement creates potential problems for the brain. The brain cannot store sugar in its cells, so it totally depends on a second-by-second fuel delivery by the blood circulating through the brain. Brain cells use 50% of all glucose in the bloodstream for fuel and 20% of all inhaled oxygen. The brain's ability to claim this large amount of glucose depends upon a bloodstream relatively free of the blood-sugar-lowering hormone, insulin; thus, the importance of chromium picolinate in the diet, as it inhibits the release of insulin.

The way to ensure adequate glucose to the brain is to avoid simple sugar foods such as candy, pastries, drinks, etc. These high-sugar foods easily and powerfully trigger insulin release. Complex carbohydrate foods such as whole grains, vegetables, nuts, peas, beans, and seeds are much more desirable and a "brain-friendly" source of sugar. They are nature's *timed-release* sugar supplements.

Each of the brain's billions of neurons functions as a microcomputer. Inside each neuron, nerve impulses are conducted electrically. However, when information exchanges from one neuron to another, the brain uses chemicals called neurotransmitters to allow brain cells to communicate with each other (chemical language).

There are approximately fifty different neurotransmitters, but the communication conducted between brain cells uses only about ten major neurotransmitters. Certain neurotransmitters carry pain sensations, while others order voluntary muscle movement; some cause excitatory emotional responses, others are inhibitory. The neurotransmitters that govern our excitatory emotional responses are called catecholamines, noradrenaline (norepinephrine) and adrenaline (epinephrine), derive from the amino acids phenylalanine and tyrosine. Our reactions to everything we encounter, the way we are stirred by a song or an old picture, angered by an argument or emotional pain inflicted by someone we love, or amused by something we see on television—all depend on the chemical language of the brain; specifically, neurotransmitters. Too much or too little of any of these substances will make us under or overreact according to the stimulus.

How we feed the brain directly affects our production of neurotransmitters. Neurotransmitters determine our mental and emotional state of well-being. Proper nutrition and supplementation can correct or enhance mind, mood, memory, and behavior.

No drug currently in wide use, medical or recreational, addresses the root of neurotransmitter problems. Drugs merely stimulate temporary excessive release of preexisting neurotransmitter stores. They do not increase production of neurotransmitters. This fact explains why drugs often lose their effect over time, with chronic use. Once preexisting neurotransmitter stores are exhausted, the drug is unable to stimulate further neurotransmitter release into the synapses between neurons. Hence, the phenomenon

The Synapse

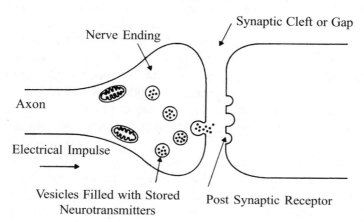

In the brain, neurotransmitters like serotonin and norepinephrine carry signals from one nerve to the next across the gap (synapse) between the two. Tryptophan enters the presynaptic nerve cell, where it converts to serotonin. As more tryptophan enters the cell, more serotonin releases into the synapse. Antidepressant drugs work by keeping more neurotransmitters in the synapse.

known as drug-abuse "crash" frequently occurs.

Greater transport into the brain of the relevant amino acids, vitamins, and minerals augment nourishment of the brain when there are less-than-adequate neurotransmitter levels. And this, in turn, requires higher levels of amino acids, vitamins, and minerals. If levels of these nutrients in the typical American junk-food diet truly and adequately promoted optimal neurotransmitter levels in the brain, we would not be seeing the epidemic level in the U.S. of antidepressant, anti-anxiety, anti-manic, anti-schizophrenic, and recreational drug use. Virtually all these drugs act either by increasing the synaptic release of brain cell neurotransmitters, without increasing their production, or by "pinch-hitting" for neurotransmitters whose synaptic levels are chronically low.

All substances of abuse either raise or lower consciousness, and deplete the available neurotransmitters needed to prevent or alleviate depressed moods. When you use drugs escape is the primary goal, you cannot escape stress, anxiety, depression, or grief. You merely prolong the healing process. Prescription drugs for stress do not restore or resolve, they *merely use available neurotransmitters.*

All major neurotransmitters are made from amino acids and from dietary protein. One of the dangers of a low-protein diet includes not producing enough amino acids to make adequate brain neurotransmitters. Apathy, lethargy, difficulty concentrating, loss of interest, and insomnia all result from not enough amino acids in the diet. ADD and hyperactive children, as well as adults, have low levels of neurotransmitters. Drug use does not produce or increase production of neurotransmitters. Drugs *only* address symptoms.

Children, as well as adults, on prolonged drug use or alcohol, have dangerously low levels of neurotransmitters. They display panic and anxiety because of the deficiency of neurotransmitters. Once proper supplementation is achieved, the symptoms of panic and anxiety decrease noticeably. You cannot restore the brain chemistry overnight by megadosing. Deficiencies must be established, then adequate amounts of amino acids, vitamins, and minerals must be implemented. All this is part of the healing process. You have taken the first step by purchasing this book.

Blood-Brain Barrier
The Protective Barrier

In 1968 Dr. Linus Pauling published an article in *Science* magazine describing the unique function of the "blood-brain barrier." Dr. Pauling postulated the brain's disadvantage in acquiring the high levels of vitamins and minerals it needs is due to the presence in the brain of a unique blood-brain barrier (B.B.B.). The B.B.B.'s major purpose is to protect the brain from water-soluble toxins. Ironically, however, most of the major brain nutrients—glucose, Vitamins B and C, minerals, and amino acids—are all water soluble. Therefore, the B.B.B. makes it difficult for the brain to absorb the large nutrients needed for delivery to other organs and tissues.

Scientific studies reported by the National Institute of Health (NIH) reveal mild nutrient deficiencies typically cause changes in mood and behavior. Other memory and mental abnormalities will present early detectable signs of nutrient deficiency. Dr. Pauling recommended an increase in the daily intake of B6, Vitamin C, and magnesium. This is far beyond R.D.A. (recommended daily allowance) levels as this produces higher blood levels of these nutrients, thus increasing their penetration of the blood-brain barrier.

Research done at M.I.T. as early as 1970 pointed to a conclusion that brain neurotransmitter levels were controlled totally by the brain, itself, independent of dietary intake of various amino acids. Further research at M.I.T. pointed to brain neurotransmitter levels are significantly influenced by a single meal. A meal rich in protein will encourage high adrenaline/norepinephrine levels with consequent high alertness and assertiveness. A meal rich in simple sugars and low in protein will usually increase brain serotonin levels. This leads to a very relaxed or even, sleepy state.

Alan Gelenberg, M.D., Department of Psychiatry at Harvard Medical School, found tyrosine to be more effective than antidepressants. Dr. Gelenberg noted that those with stress burnout and overload responded extremely well to tyrosine and B6. Tyrosine is the amino acid precursor of noradrenaline, adrenaline and dopamine.

Glutamine, one of the most plentiful amino acids in the brain, provides a major alternative fuel source for the brain with low blood-sugar levels. The amino acid, glycine, also helps alleviate sugar cravings, or that low feeling in mid afternoon. Glutamine is important as the precursor for GABA (Gamma Amino Butyric Acid). GABA and glutamine help those with problems of concentration and ADD. Glutamine also helps the brain dispose of waste ammonia, a protein breakdown byproduct irritating to the brain cells even at low levels.

Adequate vitamin and mineral intake also promotes optimum brain neurotransmitter production. B6 is essential to convert all amino acids. Pyridoxal 5' Phosphate (P5'P), the active or coenzyme form of Vitamin B6, is essential to carbohydrate, fat, and especially, protein metabolism. P5'P can be used in place of B6, is safe for children, and has no adverse side effects. The importance in providing optimal brain nutrition to facilitate optimal brain neurotransmitter production cannot be overemphasized.

Neurotransmitters are produced within neurons and stored in small packets, called *vesicles,* near the end of the neurons. People are unaware of their brain's activity. The limbic system, the feelings part of the brain, stores all fears of the past, present, and future. The GABA-receptor sites control the firing of anxiety-related messages at the cortex, the decision-making part of the brain. The brain's power plant *never shuts down and must be fed constantly.* When an electrical current flashes down the length of a neuron, neurotransmitter molecules secrete into microscopic synaptic gaps between two adjacent neurons. Once secreted into the synaptic gap, or synapse between two neurons, the enzymes in the synapse either destroy the neurotransmitters' molecules, or recycle back into the preceding neuron.

Amino Acids for Brain and Body Function

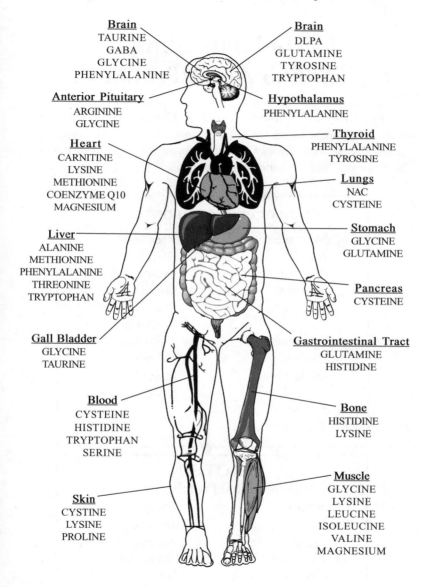

Brain
TAURINE
GABA
GLYCINE
PHENYLALANINE

Brain
DLPA
GLUTAMINE
TYROSINE
TRYPTOPHAN

Anterior Pituitary
ARGININE
GLYCINE

Hypothalamus
PHENYLALANINE

Heart
CARNITINE
LYSINE
METHIONINE
COENZYME Q10
MAGNESIUM

Thyroid
PHENYLALANINE
TYROSINE

Lungs
NAC
CYSTEINE

Liver
ALANINE
METHIONINE
PHENYLALANINE
THREONINE
TRYPTOPHAN

Stomach
GLYCINE
GLUTAMINE

Pancreas
CYSTEINE

Gall Bladder
GLYCINE
TAURINE

Gastrointestinal Tract
GLUTAMINE
HISTIDINE

Blood
CYSTEINE
HISTIDINE
TRYPTOPHAN
SERINE

Bone
HISTIDINE
LYSINE

Muscle
GLYCINE
LYSINE
LEUCINE
ISOLEUCINE
VALINE
MAGNESIUM

Skin
CYSTINE
LYSINE
PROLINE

Always add magnesium and B6 or P5'P to all amino acids.

Understanding
Amino Acids/Proteins

Proteins control almost every biochemical reaction in the body. All proteins derive from amino acids and are commonly called the *building blocks of life.* If you remove the water and fat from the body, amino acids comprise 75% of what remains.

Proteogenic Amino Acids

Nonessential	*Essential*
Alanine	Histidine
Aspartic Acid	Lysine
Arginine	Methionine
Asparagine	Phenylalanine
GABA	Threonine
Cysteine	Tryptophan
Glutamic Acid	Valine
Glutamine	Isoleucine
Proline	Leucine
Serine	
Tyrosine	

PROTEINS
Six Functional Proteins Divisions

Function	*Example*
Regulatory proteins	Hormones
Immune proteins	Immunoglobulins
Transport proteins	Hemoglobin
Contractile proteins	Muscle tissue
Structural proteins	Collagen
Enzymes	Proteinase

Source: *Interpretation Guide To Amino Acid Metabolism and Analysis,* Aatron Medical Services

All the nearly 40,000 distinct proteins found in the human body are made from only 20 amino acids called the proteogenic amino acids. Amino acids can be broken down into essential and nonessential categories. The body cannot synthesize essential amino acids; they *must* be obtained from the diet. Nonessentials can be synthesized in the body, and are not mandatory in the diet. Although the body can manufacture non-essential amino acids, an abnormality in the production of the nonessential amino acids can be detrimental metabolically. Some become conditionally essential amino acids under certain circumstances; i.e., infancy, illness, stress, etc.

Most of the protein in the body resides in the skeletal muscles. Only 0.1% of all protein is found as free amino acids. Plasma amino acids represent what is available to the body at the current time. A deficiency in one of the proteogenic amino acids can limit the body's ability to make an optimal number of certain proteins. Deficiency effects result in both health and disease.

Classification of Amino Acids

Nonessential	Conditionally Essential	Essential
Alanine	Arginine	Histidine
Asparagine	Cysteine	Isoleucine
Aspartic Acid	Cystine	Leucine
Glutamic Acid	Glutamine	Lysine
Glycine	Taurine	Methionine
Proline	Tyrosine	Phenylalanine
Serine		Threonine
		Tryptophan
		Valine

Neurotransmitters & Neuropeptides

Dr. Candace Pert is Professor of Molecular and Behavioral Science at George Washington University and formerly, Chief of the Brain Biochemistry and Clinical Neuroscience section at National Institute of Mental Health. Dr. Pert discovered the opiate, GABA, and many other peptide receptors in the brain and body. Her discoveries lead to an understanding of the chemicals that travel between the mind and body, such as neurotransmitters.

Everything in your body is being run by messenger molecules called neuropeptides or neurotransmitters. A peptide is made up of amino acids, the building blocks of proteins. Peptides are amino acids strung together very much like pearls strung in a necklace. Peptides are found throughout the brain and body. They are extremely important because they mediate intercellular communication throughout the brain and body. Dr. Pert calls neuropeptides and their receptors "the biochemical correlates of emotion."

Within the brain itself are about sixty neuropeptides. Peptides are found in the parts of the brain that mediate emotion. Neuropeptides allow the systems of the body to talk to each other. They control the opening and closing of the blood vessels in your face and throughout the body. Neuropeptides carry messages within the brain, and from the brain to all the body. Neuropeptides direct energy in the body to where it is needed the most. During times of high stress, energy must be directed not only to the brain, but to those parts of the body directly affected by the stress.

One reason the amino acid, GABA, so effectively relieves stress and anxiety is because it is able to reach the GABA receptors throughout the body and brain. Dr. Pert's research established two realms of emotion—physical and mental, found in every cell of your body. In her book, *Molecules of Emotion,* Dr. Pert states "Emotions are at the nexus between matter and mind, going back and forth between the two and influencing both." The molecular basis of our emotions are inseparable from our physiology. Part of being a healthy person means being well integrated and at peace, with all systems acting together. Neuropeptides and neurotransmitters are the keys to understanding our fear, anxiety, depression, and every emotion we feel.

The study of GABA, other amino acids, and how they affect the brain and behavior is making substantial contributions to the understanding of disease in man. Research done in the field of psychoneuroimmunology confirms disease can originate from within individuals. Major contributing factors include continuous stress overload, the environment, nutrient imbalances, and changes in brain chemistry. The immune system directly effects stress and the quality of life. The different functions of amino acids and how they affect the brain and behavior provide a major focal project for scientists and researchers.

A new age of medicine has emerged, and incorporates the substantial evidence that nutrient deficiencies can and do influence mind, mood, memory, and behavior. Amino acid requirements in the body and brain are tremendously increased by disease and inborn metabolic errors. Any time a person undergoes prolonged periods of stress, anxiety, depression, or grief, they require more amino acids; some more than others. The reason for the different requirements: biochemical individuality.

Every individual has a distinct chemical composition. The brain, glands, and bones are distinct for each person, not only in anatomy, but also in chemical composition. This does not mean that chemical compositions are fixed throughout life, or that they are not influenced by nutrition. Nutrition and amino acid deficiencies affect every tissue in the body, and most importantly, the brain.

Neurotransmitters are the brain link to smooth brain function.

Limbic System & Mental Distress Pathways

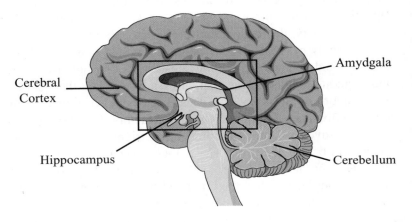

The limbic system is the region of the brain where emotion and moods are regulated and conveyed to the cerebral cortex. The limbic system contains the inhibitory neurotransmitters, GABA, glutamine, glycine, and serotonin that modulate anxiety messages in the brain. The limbic system functions as a crossover zone where signals are transmitted from the rest of the cortex into the limbic system. The limbic cortex is a link to the cerebral cortex for the control of behavior. The complex and powerful amygdala, as part of the limbic system, is the storehouse of memories, emotions, and especially traumatic experiences. Research documents the amygdala as probably functioning at birth; this accounts for negative experiences of our inner child that remain in the amygdala as unresolved anxiety, anger, and fear.

Understanding Amino Acids

Alanine

Alanine is a nonessential amino acid, and functions as an inhibitory neurotransmitter in the brain. Highest concentrations of alanine are found in the muscles. During hypoglycemia, alanine may provide an alternative source of glucose.

Elevated alanine levels in the blood can cause drug-resistant seizure disorders or severe depression. Low alanine levels are often seen with low glycine and taurine, and when the Branched Chain Amino Acids (BCAAs) are deficient. Normal alanine metabolism requires the presence of B6. Alanine is essential for the normal metabolism of tryptophan.

Best food sources for alanine include wheat germ, turkey, duck, cottage cheese, and sausage. Usual supplemental dose range is 200 to 600 mg, daily.

Arginine

Arginine, an essential amino acid, participates in many vital biochemical reactions in the brain and body, and is secreted by the anterior pituitary gland. Arginine is found in proteins consumed in the average diet, and can either be metabolized for glucose synthesis or catabolized to produce energy. Arginine performs specific and vital tasks in the body. Arginine builds muscle, enhances fat metabolism, assists in the release of growth hormone from the pituitary gland, increases sperm count and mobility in some individuals, and fights off infections.

Arginine normally constitutes approximately five to seven percent of the amino acid content of a normal, healthy, adult diet. Arginine transports via the gastrointestinal tract, and absorption occurs in the small intestine. Creatine, the high-energy supplement, forms from arginine. Creatine is used for muscle contraction, strength, and energy. Arginine is important in muscle metabolism because it provides a vehicle for transport, storage, and excretion of nitrogen. Subnormal levels of arginine are consistent with muscle weakness, fatigue, and chronic infections.

In recent years research demonstrates arginine as very beneficial to both men and women for sexual enhancement. As the primary source of nitrogen in the body, arginine is essential to production of the important biomolecule, nitric oxide (NO). Nitric oxide is present in all cells of the body. Nitric oxide forms from arginine and is a vital factor in a number of important homeostatic processes. Research indicates that nitric oxide works with arginine, and plays the major role in a male's ability to have an erection. When sexual stimulation is present, the penile nerves transmit their signals, activating the enzyme that converts arginine into nitric oxide within the penis. The release of nitric oxide triggers the erection process. Viagra cannot produce this nitric oxide.

Scientists believe that the majority of male-impotence cases are caused by poor blood flow through the patient's penis. Insufficient production of nitric oxide in the penis in males and in the vagina in females appears to be the major problem. Arginine goes beyond Viagra's capability naturally; studies at New York School of Medicine support this data.

In the best-selling book *Grow Young with HGH,* Dr. Ronald Klatz reports that Doctors A.W. Zorgniotti and E. F. Lizza gave fifteen patients 2,800 milligrams of arginine, daily, for two weeks. All had renewed sexual performance. Women who used arginine reported improved sexual responsiveness. Researchers believe arginine is effective because it is the precursor of nitric oxide. For a man, nitric oxide performs a key role in initiating and maintaining an erection. Women report increased blood flow in the vaginal area, and they test higher in production of nitric oxide.

In the immune system, nitric oxide protects the body against invading bacteria and parasites. In the brain, where nitric oxide forms in the nerve cells, it spreads in multiple directions and activates all cells in the vicinity. This activation of cells modulates multiple functions, including behavior and gastrointestinal transit flow. Nitric oxide proves vitally essential for motor learning, coordination, and long-term memory in brain function. Timothy

Maher, Ph.D., reports in his continuing education module, that angina pectoris (chest pain), atherosclerosis (hardening of the arteries), coronary artery disease, hypercholesterolemia (excessive cholesterol in the blood), hypertension, and nephrosclerosis (renal stenosis or hardening) associated with diabetes mellitus, all respond to arginine therapy.

Arginine is a very safe and effective amino acid with few side effects. However, if you have a problem with herpes (either type), take one gram of lysine daily for a week before you start taking arginine. This is necessary because arginine provides materials available for herpes replication and will cause an outbreak. Lysine blocks the replication and prevents outbreaks. If you are using arginine on an infant, are pregnant or lactating, elderly, have renal (kidney) function impairment, or have hepatic (liver) function impairment, consult a healthcare practitioner and exercise caution. Schizophrenics should use arginine with caution. Do not use arginine if you have an active malignancy, severe infection, or diabetic retinopathy.

Arginine deficiency is associated with rash, hair loss and breakage, poor wound healing, constipation, fatty liver, hepatic cirrhosis, coma, and hypoglycemia. A high content of arginine is found in meat, nuts, eggs, milk, and cheese.

Arginine, as with other amino acids, should always be taken away from mealtimes. Otherwise, amino acids compete for absorption. With proteins present in the foods, allow at least one hour before or after meals. Arginine can be combined with glutamine, ornithine, and lysine to enhance growth-hormone production.

Asparagine and Aspartic Acid

Aspartic acid is a nonessential amino acid and a major excitatory neurotransmitter. Formed in the body from glutamic acid with the presence of B6, aspartic acid plays a major role in the metabolism of ammonia via the urea cycle. Aspartic acid also metabolizes carbohydrates via the Krebs cycle, and forms constituents of DNA called pyrimidine and orotates. Asparagine forms from ATP and aspartic acid, and can convert back into aspartic acid, if needed by the body. Research indicates aspartic acid may be a stimulator of the thymus gland and the immune system.

Elevated aspartic acid levels may be seen in some patients with depression, epilepsy, stroke, high BCAAs, and low ornithine.

Good food sources of aspartic acid include meats such as pork, turkey, sausage, chicken, wheat germ, cottage and ricotta cheeses.

Branched Chain Amino Acids (BCAA)
Leucine, Isoleucine, and Valine

The branched-chain amino acids include leucine, isoleucine, and valine. As essential amino acids, BCAAs must be obtained from foods. They are especially involved in stress reactions, energy, and muscle metabolism. BCAAs are unique because the skeletal muscles use them directly as an energy source, and they promote protein synthesis.

The BCAAs are similar structurally, but have different metabolic routes. Leucine solely goes to fats; valine solely to carbohydrates; and isoleucine to both. A valine deficiency appears as neurological defects in the brain. Muscle tremors mark an isoleucine deficiency. Stress states, such as infections, trauma, surgery, fever, cirrhosis, and starvation, require proportionally more leucine than valine or isoleucine. Diseases such as hepatitis, cirrhosis, hepatic coma, or liver disease, lower the levels of BCAAs. BCAAs, as well as other amino acids, are commonly fed intravenously to chronically ill patients. The BCAAs, particularly leucine, stimulate protein synthesis, increase the re-utilization of other amino acids in many organs, and decrease protein breakdown.

As stress rises, total caloric intake needs increase, primarily due to increased protein requirements. Stress causes proteins to break down rapidly, and increases amino acid utilization three to four fold. About 30% of the diet should be protein or amino acids, especially when the body undergoes severe stress. But when taken in supplement form, BCAAs decrease the rate of amino acid and protein breakdown. More BCAAs and B6, or P5'P (Pyridoxal 5' Phosphate), are needed as stress or disease accelerates.

Use of the BCAAs by athletes, especially weight lifters, increases available energy. BCAA helps replace steroids used by those who want to build muscle mass. The BCAAs, especially leucine, greatly produce energy under many kinds of stress—from trauma, surgery, fever, infection, muscle training, and weight lifting, and for all kinds of athletic training. With prolonged exercise, about 5 to 10% of the energy used comes from amino acids, especially BCAAs. BCAAs should be used in *all* stress situations. The amount needed will depend on your physical state and stress level. Normal dosage of BCAAs is 1,000 to 3,000 mg per day, divided. *BCAAs should be taken together and not singularly.* The ingestion of only one BCAA, particularly leucine, decreases the plasma-tissue levels of valine and isoleucine.

Athletes can use BCAAs to prevent muscle breakdown. The liver does not break down the BCAAs easily, so they circulate in the body, competing for absorption against other amino acids, especially tryptophan. Brain serotonin increases with exercise, as does the ratio of BCAAs to tryptophan. Tryptophan contributes to exercise-induced fatigue, but by increasing your BCAAs during exercise, you postpone this fatigue.

At Stockholm University, during competition, researchers gave six female athletes 7.5 grams of BCAAs in a 6% carbohydrate drink. The researchers report the BCAAs increased the BCAA-to-tryptophan ratio which decreased the athletes' fatigue and increased their mental performance and focus. In another study, these researchers gave the BCAA mixture to seven cyclists. The cyclists experienced a 7% drop in their perceived exertion output and a 15% reduction in mental fatigue. The researchers concluded that the BCAAs improved athletic performance, enabled the athletes to remain more focused, reduced fatigue, and allowed more strenuous exercise.

In another study, done at Karolinska Institute in Stockholm, researchers found similar results in cross-country athletes. The researchers found comparable results to the Stockholm University study—the BCAAs serve as a source of local energy to decrease the breakdown of muscles during endurance exercises. If the BCAAs are available during exercise, they prevent the breakdown of muscle tissues while increasing protein synthesis.

BCAAs have other positive effects on the body. If you are on a reduced-calorie diet, BCAAs help you lose more weight, including more abdominal fat without altering your exercise performance. Inside the muscle cells, the BCAAs help sustain higher testosterone levels. The dosage range for BCAAs for increased athletic performance ranges from 6 to 18 grams daily, divided.

Carnitine

Carnitine was discovered in 1905 from extracts of meats, but no physiological role for carnitine could be found until fifty years later. Early research indicated carnitine to be essential to the diet, but later research discovered the body produced carnitine from lysine and methionine provided sufficient amounts of niacin, Vitamins B6, C, and iron were present. If a carnitine deficiency exists, deficiencies of lysine and methionine also exist.

Carnitine is a nonessential amino acid synthesized from lysine and methionine in the liver, kidney, and brain. Concentrations of carnitine are forty times greater in the muscles than in the plasma. Major sources of carnitine in the diet are meat, especially organ meats such as the liver, and dairy products. Vegetables, grains, and fruits contain little or no carnitine. Vegetarians are therefore more susceptible to deficiencies of carnitine, but also of lysine and methionine.

In 1973 research showed carnitine deficiencies exist in some people for various reasons. Between 1980 and 1983, almost 300 studies were published investigating carnitine's nutritional value and anomalies of carnitine metabolism causing clinical symptoms. Some carnitine deficiency symptoms include impaired lipid (fat) metabolism; lipid accumulation in the skeletal muscles, heart muscle, and liver; and progressive muscle weakness with a buildup of fats in the muscle cells. In children, carnitine deficiency may manifest as loss of muscle tone, failure to thrive, swelling in the brain, recurrent infections, hypoglycemia, and heart disturbances.

Carnitine is essential to the transportation of long-chain fatty acids into the cells where the fats can be converted to energy. Recent research indicates carnitine plays an important role in converting stored body fat into energy, energizing the heart, reducing angina attacks, controlling hypoglycemia, and is beneficial with diabetes, liver disease, and kidney disease. Carnitine primarily regulates fat burning in the body. Carnitine transports large fat molecules into the part of the cells where fats can be converted into energy. If your level of Vitamin C is low, you can have an apparent deficiency of carnitine. If carnitine is absent or deficient, many fats cannot be burned. The fats build up within the cell and bloodstream as triglycerides and cholesterol. Carnitine supplementation significantly reduces serum triglycerides and cholesterol levels, while increasing HDL (high density lipids or good cholesterol). Dosages are 1,000 to 3,000 mg per day, divided.

Normal cardiac function is dependent on adequate amounts of carnitine. In angina, carnitine helps improve oxygen utilization and energy metabolism by the heart muscle. By improving the fat utilization and energy production, carnitine prevents the buildup of toxic fatty acid metabolites. These metabolites can cause cell-membrane damage throughout the heart, contributing to impaired heart-muscle contraction, arrhythmias (irregular beats), and death of the heart muscle. Carnitine supplementation helps prevent the production of these fatty acid metabolites.

Many clinical trials have shown that carnitine improves angina and heart disease, and is beneficial in recovery from a heart attack, arrhythmias, and congestive heart failure. Oral supplementation with carnitine helps normalize heart carnitine levels, thereby allowing the heart to use its limited oxygen supply more efficiently. In one study, patients released from the hospital received 4 grams of carnitine daily, and recovered more quickly from their heart attacks. They showed dramatic improvements in heart rate, blood pressure, rhythm disturbances, angina attacks, and clinical signs of impaired heart function compared to the control group.

Carnitine increases heart rate, pressure rate, heart-pacing duration, and decreases left ventricular and diastolic pressures. It increases muscle strength, and is beneficial to heart patients by increasing exercise endurance at doses of 20 to 40 mg/kg (1,400 to 2,800 mg/day). Other studies indicate that carnitine lowers the exercise heart rate, and extends the time of exercise prior to the onset of angina at doses of 40 mg/kg (about 2,800 mg in 150 pound individuals). Carnitine proves very beneficial in congestive heart patients.

Intermittent claudication is intermittent pain in the calf muscle. This is often described as a cramp or tightness causing pain in the calf, much like angina occurs in the heart. Carnitine improves distances walked without pain in intermittent claudication and other peripheral vascular diseases. In one study, 2 grams of carnitine, twice daily, showed a 75% increase in the walking distance after three weeks of supplementation. This results from the improved energy metabolism within the muscle.

In patients with uremia or kidney disease, carnitine may reduce the risk factor for atherosclerosis and coronary heart disease. Carnitine dramatically reduces triglycerides and cholesterol levels, while increasing HDL (good cholesterol) levels. In addition, carnitine reduces muscle cramping and muscle weakness by restoring muscle carnitine levels. Carnitine deficiencies usually exist in hemodialysis patients due to decreased carnitine synthesis.

Diabetics have reduced blood levels of carnitine. Since cardiovascular disease and reduced kidney and liver function are found in diabetics, supplementing with carnitine is encouraged.

Reduced levels of carnitine in skeletal muscles are seen in patients with various muscular dystrophies. The muscular weaknesses experienced by these patients is believed to result from the low carnitine levels. Carnitine supplementation increases muscle strength, while decreasing lipid levels.

Carnitine also plays an important role in the production of heat in brown fat. The "brown fat" helps us acclimate to cold temperatures, and is thought to help determine how much of the food eaten is burned for heat, and how much is stored as body fat. During poor-weight loss diets, carnitine prevents the accumulation of ketones in the blood stream. Ketosis can be life threatening, if uncontrolled. And ketonic states can cause the loss of potassium, magnesium, and calcium.

In cancer patients receiving chemotherapy, carnitine has been shown to protect the heart during adriamycin chemotherapy. Additionally, carnitine helps alleviate some of the toxicity associated with chemotherapy through its effect on the mitochondrial integrity.

Carnitine helps improve the symptoms attributed to anticonvulsant medications such as Valproic acid (Depakote, Depakene) and carbamezepine (Tegretol and Epitol). Carnitine may offer protection against drug toxicity.

Recent studies indicate carnitine may be a factor with depression. Supplementation with 1,000 mg per day, divided, is helpful.

But carnitine supplementation does not need to be limited to people with cardiovascular problems. Effective utilization of fatty acids by the heart and skeletal muscles depends upon ample supplies of carnitine. Supplementation with 1 to 2 grams, two to three times daily, results in significant improvements in cardiovascular function in response to exercise, especially endurance related activities. It may benefit healthy people as well as athletes by helping burn certain amino acids, called BCAAs or branch chain amino acids in the skeletal muscles. During fasting or prolonged strenuous exercise, the BCAAs provide a significant amount of metabolic energy. Ketones result from the incomplete burning of fat, and are extremely toxic to the nervous system and brain. Carnitine helps to significantly lower the ketone levels.

The daily dose of carnitine ranges between 1,000 to 4,000 mg in divided doses. Carnitine is very safe with no significant side effects ever reported in any human studies. But use *only* the L-carnitine form of carnitine. There are no know adverse interactions between carnitine and any drug or nutrient. When carnitine and coenzyme Q10 are combined, they appear to work synergistically.

Cysteine and Cystine

Cysteine is the considered conditionally essential, and is one of the sulfur-containing amino acids. Cystine is the stable form of cysteine. Conversion of one to the other occurs in the body, as either is needed. If Vitamin C is not present, cysteine converts to cystine. Research now focuses on the protective role of dietary amino acids. Cysteine builds proteins, such as those in hair, and also helps destroy harmful chemicals in the body such as acetaldehyde and free radicals produced by smoking and drinking.

Cysteine spares methionine (another important amino acid) and can completely replace dietary methionine if the diet is supplemented by appropriate amounts of folic acid and Vitamin B12. Cysteine resides abundantly in proteins such as keratin in hair (12%) and trypsinogen (10%). Cysteine acts is a detoxifier. Heavy metals such as mercury, lead, and cadmium will be "tied up" by cysteine so it can be removed from the body.

Cysteine may protect heavy drinkers and smokers against acetaldehyde poisoning from chronic alcohol intake or smoking, according to Dr. Herbert Sprince at the V.A. Hospital in Coatesville, Pennsylvania, and Thomas Jefferson University in Philadelphia.

Pearson reports cysteine is effective "not only in preventing hangovers, but also in preventing brain and liver damage from alcohol, and in preventing damage such as emphysema and cancer caused by smoking." Cysteine has been found to offer a degree of protection against radiation.

Recently, Dr. William Philpott postulated that cysteine is necessary for the utilization of Vitamin B6. His studies suggest "a majority of chronic degenerative illnesses, whether physical or mental, have a Vitamin B6 utilization disorder. The culprit causing this Vitamin B6 utilization problem seems to be cysteine deficiency." Dr. Philpott recommends patients having the Vitamin B6 utilization problem take 1.5 grams of L-cysteine three times a day for a month, and then reduce it to twice a day. Vitamin C should always be taken with cysteine.

A specialized cysteine known as NAC, or N-Acetyl Cysteine, was first produced by Mead Johnson for the treatment of excess mucus. The primary use for NAC is as a mucus-reducing agent. Mucus strands are broken up to decrease viscosity and congestion associated with excess mucus and sinus drainage. Oral supplementation of NAC is used with allergies, bronchitis, chronic sinusitis, asthma, pneumonia, cystic fibrosis, and even the common cold. NAC modulates the production of, and the precursor to, glutathione. In turn, glutathione helps protect the body against natural and man-made oxidants. Glutathione is an antitoxin and a neurotransmitter. Supplemental NAC dosage is usually 600 mg, twice to three times daily.

Diabetics should not use cysteine because it can cause glucose levels to change.

GABA

The Anxiety Amino Acid

GABA (Gamma Amino Butyric Acid), an inhibitory neurotransmitter, is found throughout the central nervous system (CNS). GABA assumes an ever-enlarging role as a significant influence on pain, stress, anxiety, and depression as well as stress-induced illnesses. By January 1998, there were over 3,000 documents and texts on GABA, describing how it affects anxiety/stress in the brain.

Dr. Eugene Roberts discovered GABA in 1950. Dr. Roberts established that GABA was involved in the conditions of nerve impulses and had widespread distribution throughout the brain and body. In the early 1970s, Dr. Candace Pert, a pharmacologist, discovered GABA receptor sites throughout the brain and body. Dr. Pert's research demonstrates the importance of GABA in the stress-anxiety network.

Of all the brain synapses 40 to 50% of the synapses contain GABA. GABA is the most widely distributed neurotransmitter in the brain and plays a vital role in neuronal and behavioral inhibition. GABA is present in a concentration some 200 to 1000 times greater than neurotransmitters such as acetylcholine, norepinephrine, and 5-HTP. The highest concentration of GABA resides in the basal ganglia followed by the hypothalamus, hippocampus, cortex, amygdala, and thalamus.

If you examine a step-by-step process of what happens in the brain when you feel stress and anxiety, you would see how GABA works to slow down messages. Panic, anxiety, or stress-related messages begin to release numerous signals, and concurrently a physiological response begins to take place—the fight-or-flight syndrome.

The unceasing alert signals from the limbic system eventually overwhelm the cortex (the decision-making part of the brain), and the ability of the cortex and the rest of the stress network becomes exhausted. The balance between the limbic system, and in fact, the rest of the brain to communicate in an orderly manner depends critically on inhibition. GABA inhibits the cells from firing, diminishing the anxiety-related messages from reaching the cortex.

GABA fills certain receptor sites in the brain and body. This slows down and blocks the excitatory levels of the brain cells that are about to receive the anxiety-related, incoming message. When the message is received by the cortex, it does not overwhelm you with anxiety, panic or pain. You are able to maintain control and remain calm. But, if you are under prolonged stress or anxiety, your brain exhausts all the available GABA and other inhibitory neurotransmitters, thus allowing anxiety, fear, panic and pain to attack you from every direction. Your ability to reason diminishes. In a full blown anxiety or panic attack, physical symptoms include excessive sweating, trembling, muscle tension, weakness, loss of control, disorientation, difficulty breathing, constant fear, headaches, diarrhea, depression, and unsteady legs.

Research done at the Pain & Stress Center, in San Antonio, with patients suffering from all types of stress, pain, muscle spasms or anxiety/panic attacks, demonstrated pure GABA, 375 or 750 mg, can mimic the tranquilizing effects of Valium or Librium *without* the possibility of addiction or fear of being sedated. GABA fills the receptor in the brain and nourishes the brain with what should be there. Pure GABA dissolves in water, and is tasteless and odorless. The calming effect usually occurs within 10 to 12 minutes.

Tranquilizers provide only temporary relief. We have seen many patients on Xanax that still experience anxiety. They have been told it is not addicting—it is! *THERE IS NO SUCH THING AS A TRANQUILIZER DEFICIENCY!* Nutrient deficiencies can and do change behavior. Human behavior involves the functioning of the whole nervous system, and the nervous system requires amino acids. GABA, glutamine, and glycine proves vital for energy and the smooth running of brain functions.

B6 (pyridoxine) and Mag Link (magnesium chloride) are GABA's most important partners. We have successfully used GABA, glutamine, and glycine with patients to ease anxiety, muscle pain/ spasms, and nervous stomachs. GABA 375 or 750 are freeform, not combined with anything else. There is a GABA with niacinamide and inositol on the market, but let me caution you—*do not megadose*, with this form. If you do, you will have side effects. Side effects include tingling lips and extremities, rapid heart beat, shortness of breath, flushing, nausea, and increased anxiety. If this occurs, drink 16 ounces of water, and eat a couple of soda crackers. If you weigh less than 125 pounds, use GABA 375, or *one-half* of a GABA 750 capsule.

Special Note: Magnesium is the stress mineral, and is involved in over 300 enzyme reactions in the body. Take magnesium along with B6. The best form for maximum absorption and tolerance is magnesium chloride (Mag Link). Magnesium chloride is the same form of magnesium present in the body.

Glutamic Acid

Glutamic acid is a nonessential amino acid which can be synthesized by the body, or be converted into glutamine and GABA. Glutamic acid or glutamate is thought to be an excitatory neurotransmitter. It acts as a brain ammonia detoxifier.

Since glutamic acid can be manufactured from aspartic acid, ornithine, arginine, proline, and alpha-ketoglutarate, no deficiencies of glutamic acid have ever been seen. Elevation of glutamic acid may be present in some schizophrenics, epileptics, and patients with gout. In fact, epileptics generally have an elevation of glutamic and aspartic acids, and have low levels of GABA, taurine, and glycine.

Rich food sources of glutamic acid include sausage, ham, bacon, yogurt, turkey, chicken, duck, cottage cheese, wheat germ, and granola.

Glutamine

Glutamine, a conditionally essential amino acid, is the third most abundant amino acid in the blood and brain. Glutamine, an inhibitory neurotransmitter acts as a precursor for GABA, the antianxiety amino acid. Glutamine crosses the blood-brain-barrier into the brain, where it increases energy and mental alertness. It helps the brain dispose of waste ammonia, a protein breakdown byproduct. Ammonia irritates brain cells, even at low levels. Recent scientific research demonstrates its link to the most important functions of the body's vital organs and musculoskeletal system. Glutamine assists the body in muscle development when illness causes muscle wasting—sometimes seen following a high fever, chronic stress, illness, or a traumatic accident. Glutamine provides a major alternative fuel source for the brain with low blood sugar levels.

In 1980 glutamine was reestablished as a conditionally essential amino acid; prior to 1980 glutamine was considered a nonessential amino acid. A conditionally essential amino acid means that under normal circumstances, the body can make (synthesize) adequate quantities of that amino acid; but in times of stress such as fever, illness, trauma, dieting, or chemotherapy, the body cannot make as much as it requires. An additional amount of the amino acid must be taken in nutrient form to prevent a deficiency.

Glutamine's most important function is strengthening the immune system. Glutamine supports the multiplication of selected white cells which strengthen the body's defense system. Glutamine aids other immune cells in killing bacteria, healing wounds, and maintaining and supporting glutathione, as an important antioxidant. Glutamine also supports pancreatic growth.

Scientists at NIH in 1970 found glutamine to be the most important nutrient for the intestinal tract. During times of illness, the body uses more glutamine to help tissue repair in the kidneys, intestines, and liver. For many years glutamine was considered a nonessential amino acid, but research over the past several years brought forth a wave of new, important information to change this view.

Every day researcher conduct more studies on the healing power of amino acids. Glutamine deserves special attention. Studies show glutamine supplementation during cancer treatment increased the effectiveness of many chemotherapy drugs, and increased tumor kill-off. Systemic infections (sepsis) decreased by up to 80% with glutamine supplementation. The mechanisms appear to be increased intestinal integrity and reduced intestinal ulcerations. Glutamine decreased weight loss and increased nitrogen balance. Following radiation, glutamine decreased mortality to the point of ameliorating toxicity. Additionally, glutamine augmented healing of radiated intestines.

Some amino acids help the body resist the effects of the radiation which is becoming a significant pollutant and potentially, a worldwide problem. In cancer patients, glutamine enhances the effectiveness of chemotherapy and radiation treatments, while reducing the toxicity and damage to the body. Dosages vary in amounts, but a rule of thumb is 0.5 grams/kilogram of body weight daily. For best results, take glutamine prior to treatment and continue throughout therapy. Research has shown glutamine is the second-most important fuel for the cells' lining in the colon.

The main nutrient needed for intestinal repair is glutamine. Leaky-gut syndrome is recognized more often today due to the increased use of anti-inflammatory medications such as Motrin, Advil, Ibuprofen, Dolobid, Anaprox, Orudis, Naprosyn, etc. Leaky-gut syndrome makes the intestines more permeable and allows substances and foods which do not normally pass into the circulation to cross. Food allergies can result, causing more discomfort and pain. But glutamine helps the gut to heal and makes the intestines less permeable. Japanese researchers found glutamine helps stomach ulcers heal. In the book *The Ultimate Nutrient, Glutamine,* Judy Shabert reports that Douglas Wilmore, M.D. of Harvard Medical School found glutamine is a key to the metabolism and maintenance of muscle. Glutamine is the primary energy source for the immune system and factors that are enhanced by growth hormone.

Glutamine helps clear the body of waste through the kidneys and liver. For those with impending surgery, glutamine supplements should be considered before, during, and after surgery. New research demonstrates the body's release of amino acids during times of stress includes one-third in the form of glutamine. Further research revealed the muscles synthesize glutamine as they break down in times of heavy stress. When glutamine was taken with balanced amino acids, muscle breakdown (atrophy) was essentially prevented. Glutamine is an effective growth hormone stimulator according to Vincent Giampapa, M.D., Director at the Longevity Institute International. In the book *Grow Young with HGH,* Dr. Giampapa reported that two grams of glutamine are more potent than one gram of arginine, ornithine, and lysine combined.

Note: Over the past years there has been confusion regarding glutamine, glutamic acid, and glutamate. Glutamine is not glutamic acid, glutamate, MSG, or glutathione. Glutamine, GABA, and glycine are rapidly becoming the most important therapeutic amino acids of the twenty-first century.

Neurotransmitters in Brain Function

The amino acid trio of glutamine, GABA, and glycine, along with Vitamin B6, the cofactor, represent the major inhibitory neurotransmitters in the brain. Glutamine is found in the nerves of the hippocampus—the memory center of the brain, in the cranial nerves, and in many other areas of the brain. These three amino acids work together, and are inhibitory neurotransmitters. Anyone taking amino acids must take Vitamin B6 to metabolize these amino acids.

Glutamine studies reported intellectually impaired children and adults demonstrated an increase in IQ after taking glutamine in combination with ginkgo and Vitamin B6. Research done by Dr. Roger Williams at the University of Texas, Clayton Foundation, showed children and adults classified ADHD showed a marked improvement when taking glutamine, 250 mg to 1,000 mg, daily. Dosage depends on age and weight. At the Pain & Stress Center we use a Balanced Neurotransmitter Complex plus GABA, along with AC (Anxiety Control 24). If needed, extra glutamine powder and ginkgo are added. Results have been excellent. The Balanced Neurotransmitter Complex formula assists brain communication and allows the brain cells to talk to each other. Recent discoveries found 50 or 60 neuropeptides in the immune system, as well as in the brain. Each unique neuropeptide has its own receptor. These intercellular neuropeptides and receptors mediate communication among the brain, glands, and immune system. Neuropeptides are peptides made up of amino acids, the building blocks of proteins. Neuropeptides and their receptors form the biochemical correlates of emotion.

GABA and glutamine are found not *only* in the brain, but in the receptor sites throughout the body. Amino acids can and do change mind, mood, memory, and behavior. A particular herb, Ginkgo Biloba demonstates excellent results in enhancing concentration. Ginkgo increases blood flow to the head, and improves mental functioning and the ability to focus for longer periods of time. Ginkgo has also been helpful after a stroke by increasing circulation to the brain. In his book *Herbal Tonic Therapies,* Daniel Mowrey, Ph.D. reviews studies using Ginkgo. In one study patients received 120 mg of ginkgo, daily, for twelve weeks. Patients reported a definite improvement in alertness and memory.

Ginkgo and glutamine provide an effective combination for those with problems in concentration, memory, and staying on task. Ginkgo promotes an increased nerve transmission rate, and improves synthesis and turnover of brain neurotransmitters.

For those with alcohol cravings, Dr. Roger Williams pioneering in glutamine research found 3,000 to 4,000 milligrams of glutamine, daily, will stop the craving for alcohol and decrease the craving for sweets. Since pure pharmaceutical glutamine, such as Super Glutamine, is tasteless, and mixes readily with water or any cool liquid, patients find it easy to take. Patients also reported a lift from fatigue, both mental and physical. One alcoholic stopped drinking when glutamine was administered daily. Two years later the patient was still free from the craving for alcohol. He maintained a nutritional support program. Dr. Lorene Rogers, researcher at the University of Texas, Clayton Foundation, reported several cases in which glutamine was successful and placebos ineffective. Glutamine was given to one group of alcoholics and placebos to the other. The group taking at least 3,000 milligrams of glutamine daily were free of alcohol craving.

The brain converts glutamine to energy, and with glutamine the brain's main fuel, it converts the glutamine to GABA, with the help of magnesium. Without continued high energy in the brain, the rest of the mind and body will NOT function properly. The brain requires a huge supply of glucose and oxygen in order to perform properly. This energy supply transports via the bloodstream. Proper circulation ensures the brain has the glutamine (energy) it needs.

Unfortunately, foods are not a good source of glutamine. The foods highest in glutamine include meat, chicken, and eggs, but in the *raw* form. Cooking or heating inactivates glutamine, so your best source is supplement form.

Glutamine is available in capsule and powder forms. If using powder form, put in *cool* water or juice. Heat destroys glutamine.

Glycine

Glycine is a nonessential amino acid, and has the simplest structure of all the amino acids resembling glucose (blood sugar) and glycogen (excess sugar converted in the liver for storage). Glycine is sweet to taste, and can be used as a sweetener. It can mask bitterness and saltiness. Pure glycine dissolves readily in water. As the third major inhibitory neurotransmitter in the brain glycine readily passes the blood-brain barrier. The body needs glycine for the formation of DNA, collagen, phospholipids, and for the release of energy.

According to Ronald Kotulak in his book, *Inside the Brain,* glycine "helps trigger brain cells to fire electric charges and speed learning." Glycine helps spasticity and seizures, and is involved in behaviors related to convulsions and retinal function. If is taken orally, glycine increases the urinary excretion of uric acid, and is possibly a useful adjunct to gout.

Glycine is an essential intermediate in the metabolism of protein, peptides, and bile salts. Liver detoxification compounds, such as glutathione, must have glycine present for formation. Glycine removes heavy metals such as lead from the body, and also decreases the craving for sugar. In many cases, replacing sugar on foods such as cereal. Glycine has been shown to calm aggression in both, children and adults. When combined with GABA and glutamine, glycine influences brain function by slowing down anxiety-related messages from the limbic system. Glycine is effective in alcohol withdrawal as it decreases the craving for sugar.

As a very nontoxic amino acid, glycine can be used by both children and adults. Glycine is found in high concentrations in meats and wheat germ.

Usual dosage range is 500 to 3,000 mg, per day, in divided doses.

Histidine

Histidine, one of the essential amino acid, is required in large amounts in infants. Histidine is necessary for the maintenance of myelin sheaths of nerves, has vasodilating and mild anti-inflammatory properties. The neurotransmitter, histamine, derives from histidine. Histidine promotes large increases in brain histamine content, especially in the hypothalamus.

People with abnormally high amounts of histamine often demonstrate a history of psychiatric problems ranging from mild to severe. People with chronic pain and fibromyalgia demonstrate high histamine levels represented by joint swelling. High histidine and histamine levels are often seen in patients with obsessive-compulsive disorders, depression, and phobias. Low blood-histamine levels are found with rheumatoid arthritis and Parkinson's disease.

Best food sources for histidine include pork, wheat germ, sausage, chicken, turkey, duck, ricotta cheese, and cottage cheese.

Lysine

Lysine is an essential amino acid, and must be obtained by the diet, as it cannot be produced by the human body. In the body, lysine is a critical protein required for growth, tissue repair, and production of hormones, enzymes, and antibodies. Additionally, it helps reduce the incidence of herpes outbreaks.

Symptoms of lysine deficiency include fatigue, inability to concentrate, irritability, bloodshot eyes, retarded growth, anemia, hair loss, and reproductive problems.

Lysine is effective against herpes because it reduces viral growth. It suppresses the virus by restoring the balance of nutrients retarding viral growth. The proper balance of lysine to arginine ratio helps suppress the virus. (See section on herpes.)

Good food sources of lysine include eggs, meat, fish, milk, cheese, and yeast. Cereals, rice, millet, wheat, and sesame seeds contain very little lysine. Amounts required for optimum health varies widely from person to person from 500 to 1,600 mg per day, depending on their particular biochemistry. If outbreaks of herpes occur, increase the amount to 3,000 mg, daily, until outbreak subsides.

Methionine

Methionine, an essential amino acid, represents one of the sulfur containing amino acids. Methionine is a methyl donor, critical for the formation of many important substances such as nucleic acids, epinephrine, choline, lecithin, carnitine, melatonin, collagen, serine, creatine, and deanol. Additionally, methionine can be a detoxifying agent assisting the removal from the body of heavy metals such as lead. Methionine is necessary for selenium to be absorbed and utilized in the body. As an antioxidant, it helps protect the body from effects of radiation. Normal metabolism of homocysteine require B6 and methionine. Excess homocysteine can cause plaque formation in the arteries, leading to cardiovascular disease. If supplementing with methionine, *always add B6 and folic acid* to prevent a buildup of homocysteine. Methionine can be synthesized into cysteine, cystine, and taurine, if sulfur is present.

Excess methionine has been suggested in one type of schizophrenia, while low levels are seen with depression. Supplementing with methionine helps lower histamine levels in the body, and sufferers of allergies, asthma, and chronic pain may find methionine supplementation helpful. Heroin addicts often have low pain thresholds and high histamine levels. Methionine helps lower the excess histamine levels usually present during heroin, amphetamine, or barbiturate withdrawal. In some depressed patients, methionine lifts depression with supplementation of 1 gram of methionine, morning and evening. Compared to MAO-inhibitor antidepressants, methionine proves more effective.

Good food sources for methionine include sunflowers, pork, sausage, duck, wild game, lentils, pumpkin and sesame seeds, avocado, cottage cheese, cheese, and wheat germ.

SAMe
S-AdenosylMethionine

Recently, reports about SAMe (S-adenosylmethionine) abound for the treatment of depression. SAMe became commercially available in the U.S. in 1999. SAMe derives from methionine and adenosine triphosphate (ATP). The compound of SAMe is *very unstable* and requires refrigeration from the manufacturing phase to the finished capsule in the bottle.

Oral absorption of SAMe is *less than one percent,* so it is not very bioavailable to the body. In one study, only 71% of the patients treated with oral SAMe increased their serum SAMe concentrations. Most studies done with SAMe used the parenteral (injection) form.

Patients with a history of mania, or bipolar disorder, should not use SAMe. Also, the safety of its use by heart or coronary patients remains questionable. SAMe transforms into homocysteine. It is unknown if SAMe increases the homocysteine levels in the body or influences the development of heart disease. Side effects from SAMe include nausea, mania, forced speech, and the display of grandiose ideas. Dr. Phyllis Bronson of the Aspen Clinic, reports that some patients feel extremely irritable because SAMe impacts their levels of dopamine. She advises patients to work with their individual biochemistry. Individuals with high serum methionine (per amino acid analysis), taking psychotropic (such as thorazine or haldol) or SSRI (Selective Serotonin Reuptake Inhibitors) medications, may experience temporary psychosis or extreme agitation after taking SAMe.

The dosage of SAMe is usually 800 mg, twice daily, taken on an empty stomach. SAMe is very expensive compared to other supplements and drugs. The average cost of a month's supply of SAMe is $250. At the Pain & Stress Center, combining BNC (Balanced Neurotransmitter Complex®) with methionine proves more effective than SAMe. This better-than-SAMe combination is stable and much less expensive for the treatment of depression. If you combine methionine with BNC, you will supply your brain with all the neurotransmitters it needs to make SAMe. Your body knows how much SAMe is right for you and will manufacture all the SAMe it needs. If you weigh less than 150 pounds, use two BNC in the morning and 1500 milligrams of methionine, twice daily. If you weigh more than 150 pounds, use two BNC capsules in the morning and afternoon, along with 1500 mg methionine, twice daily. Add 150 mg of timed-release B6, to activate the amino acids.

Phenylalanine

Phenylalanine, an essential amino acid, functions as the parent substance, or precursor of tyrosine. Phenylalanine converts to tyrosine in the liver.

Phenylalanine Pathway

Phenylalanine → Tyrosine → Dopamine →Norepinephrine → Epinephrine

Phenoketonurics (PKU) cannot convert phenylalanine into tyrosine because PKUs lack the enzyme, phenylalanine hydroxylase.

The formation of the hormone, thyroid, requires phenylalanine. Although phenylalanine is not found in the brain, it resides in many brain peptides, proteins, and neurotransmitters. Phenylalanine is the raw substance that produces several compounds of the catecholamine family responsible for the transmission of nerve impulses, assuming an adequate supply of phenylalanine. Norepinephrine, a major neurotransmitter, derives from tyrosine or phenylalanine. The amount of norepinephrine available to the brain is predisposed by the amount of phenylalanine or tyrosine available. Phenylalanine is one of the few amino acids readily converted into brain compounds like norepinephrine that control a person's mood. Phenylalanine or tyrosine, helps give a positive, uplifting effect on mood, alertness, and ambition. Often, this amino acid is deficient in depressed people. Phenylalanine can also stimulate the release of CCK (cholecystokinin), that in effect, turns off the appetite.

Other phenylalanine derivatives such as epinephrine are excreted at the nerve terminals in the hypothalamus, and norepinephrine is excreted at the sympathetic nerve endings, giving rise to the fight-or-flight response. Norepinephrine is stored in presynaptic vesicles in certain central synapses. During times of stress, the body's adrenal glands are under immense pressure to produce epinephrine and norepinephrine. Often, they become low or depleted. This depletion can lead to depression and stress which can cause pain, anxiety, uncertainty, and fear.

Supplementing with phenylalanine or tyrosine helps to increase the level of norepinephrine in the brain. Many antidepressants work by increasing or manipulating the norepinephrine level in the brain. Often the drugs work by blocking the norepinephrine from re-entering the vesicles or pouches found at the synapse. The natural way to normalize the brain levels of norepinephrine is with supplementation of tyrosine or phenylalanine. Therapeutic dosage ranges from 500 to 1,500 mg per day. Phenylalanine should be used with extreme caution in hypertensive patients; and always take with food. People taking MAO inhibitors or tricyclic antidepressants should not use phenylalanine or tyrosine.

The DL-form of phenylalanine, or DLPA, was found to be effective in the treatment of pain, and for the depression resulting from the pain. DLPA increases the production of PEA, norepinephrine, and endorphins. PEA is a neurotransmitter-type substance with structural resemblance to amphetamine, a stimulant drug. Endorphins are the morphine-like neurotransmitters that decrease pain and gives a sense of well-being. DLPA increases endorphins by preventing the breakdown of the endorphins in the brain, so they remain there longer. If you use DLPA, the suggested amount is 750 mg, four times daily.

Food sources of phenylalanine include dairy products such as cottage cheese, milk, other cheeses; meats such as chicken, turkey, and duck; and pecans, sesame seeds, lima beans, and lentils.

Therapeutic dosages of DLPA range from 500 to 3,000 mg per day, divided.

Proline

As a nonessential amino acid, proline is required for the formation of collagen; but Vitamin C must be present. The body can manufacture proline from ornithine or glutamic acid and, if needed, the body convert back into orthinine.

Elevation of proline may be found in alcoholics with cirrhosis, and in some patients with depression or seizure disorders. Convulsions, elevated blood calcium levels, and osteoporosis may be caused by excess proline from a genetic error.

Good food sources of proline include cottage and ricotta cheeses, eggs, pork, luncheon meats, wheat germ, turkey, and duck.

Supplemental dose ranges from 500 to 1,000 mg, with Vitamin C.

Serine

Serine, a nonessential amino acid, is synthesized from glycine with the presence of folic acid and B6. Serine is involved in DNA synthesis. Serine, in combination with carbohydrates, may form glycoproteins. As an immunosuppressive, serine may possibly be helpful in auto-immune diseases. Serine is required for the formation of choline, ethanolamine, phospholipids and sarcosine necessary for the formation of neurotransmitters, and to stabilize cell membranes. Phospholipids are made from phosphatidylserine, and requires the presence of methionine and folic acid. Excess serine may cause psychosis and elevation of blood pressure.

Phosphatidylserine (PS) is a component of brain cell membranes. Studies support phosphatidylserine's importance in brain functions such as memory and alertness, as well as enhanced function of the aging brain. Often, aging involves alteration of structure and biochemical changes within the brain. These can include changes in neuronal membrane lipid makeup and enzyme activity, reduced production and metabolism of neurotransmitters, and loss of nerve synaptic connections. In one study, 35 patients (19 males and 16 females) with prevalent involvement of mental functions associated with behavioral changes, were treated with PS (300 mg, daily) for a period of two months. The therapeutic activity of PS was evaluated through neuropsychological tests and behavioral rating scales. Results demonstrated PS was a beneficial treatment for mild to moderate deterioration of cognitive function. Another study involved probable Alzheimer's disease patients. The study confirmed that PS treated patients improved several cognitive functions; and suggested early stage Alzheimer patients may benefit most from PS supplementation with a dosage of 100 mg, three times, daily.

Good food sources include cottage and ricotta cheeses, wheat, wheat germ, pork, luncheon meat, turkey, sausage, peanuts, and soy.

Taurine

Taurine is now classified as a conditionally essential amino acid in the adult; but in infants and children, taurine is an essential amino acid and must be obtained from the diet for normal brain development. In the developing brain, the concentration of taurine is four times that of the adult brain. Some scientists hypothesize that taurine deficiency may cause sudden-infant-death syndrome.

Taurine is a major inhibitory, sulfur amino acid. Research

demonstrates these substances are involved in the functions of the cerebral cortex, cerebellum, hippocampus, hypothalamus, and in spinal and retinal neurons. Taurine in the adult is synthesized from cysteine and methionine, provided B6 and some zinc are present. Taurine is found throughout the body abundantly in the heart muscle, olfactory bulb, central nervous system, and brain—specifically the hippocampus and pineal gland. Taurine participates in a multitude of functions in the body involving the gallbladder, brain, heart, eyes, and vascular systems. As a major inhibitory amino acid, taurine's structure closely resembles the structure and metabolism of the other inhibitory neurotransmitters, GABA and glycine.

In the heart, taurine is the most concentrated amino acid. Taurine modulates heart muscular contractility and rhythms. Taurine plays a part in calcium metabolism in the heart. Taurine affects the admission of calcium into the heart-muscle cells where it is necessary for nerve impulses (heart rhythms). Some studies suggest taurine may increase the survival rate after a heart attack and reduce the elevation of calcium content in both aorta and heart muscles. The regulation of calcium may prevent the progression of arteriosclerosis.

When the body experiences chronic stress, the concentration of taurine increases in the heart. After a heart attack, the levels of taurine often decrease dramatically. In some cases, the levels drop to one-third the normal. The loss of intracellular taurine may contribute to arrhythmias (abnormal heartbeats) where acute ischemia (low oxygen levels within the heart muscle) occurs. In Japan, doctors are using taurine widely for all types of heart disease. When congestive heart failure occurs, the concentration of taurine increases as the body tries to naturally correct the problem metabolically. In one study, congestive heart failure (CHF) patients were given 4 grams of taurine, per day, for a month. Nineteen of the 24 patients improved. Another double-blind crossover study involved fourteen patients. The patients were given 6 grams of taurine, or a placebo, in additional to conventional treatment in a randomized crossover design for four weeks, with a two-week washout period in-between. Eleven of the fourteen or 78% improved on taurine compared to twenty-one percent, or three of fourteen, on the placebo. While on the placebo, the heart-failure scores did not change appreciably, but the heart-failure scores decreased significantly for the patients on taurine. Additionally, during the taurine administration, no patient worsened, whereas four placebo patients did get worse.

Taurine seems to assist in CHF by acting as a diuretic, ridding the body of excess water and sodium, and as a heart stimulator with doses of 2 grams per day. Taurine and magnesium levels drop dramatically whenever heart arrhythmias occur, and replenishing both assists in controlling heart arrhythmias. Taurine helps prevent the decrease of potassium within the cells of the heart. Decreased potassium can cause electrical instability, leading to heart arrhythmias. Additionally, taurine helps balance the calcium and potassium levels in the heart.

Normal brain development in infants requires taurine. It protects and stabilizes the brain's fragile cell membranes. Taurine acts as an inhibitory neurotransmitter in the brain, like the neurotransmitters, GABA and glycine. In the brain, the site of greatest seizure activity, researchers found low taurine concentrations. Taurine proves effective in the treatment of epilepsy, acting as an anticonvulsant. The levels are lower than normal for over half of the amino acids, if epilepsy is present; but the levels of taurine are higher than normal, except in the cerebrospinal fluid. The usual dosage of taurine for epilepsy is 3,000 mg, per day, with a non-protein meal. Taurine helps people with tics or other spastic conditions. As a word of caution, taurine should not be taken simultaneously with aspirin or any salicylates.

In patients with tics, twitches, or spastic conditions, taurine proves helpful. In her book, *Tired or Toxic*, Dr. Sherry Rogers reports the tics of Tourette's syndrome as abnormal *firings* of the nervous system. Research on Tourette's points to multiple triggers, but taurine assists in reducing the tics. The usual dosage for tics is 1,000 mg, twice to three times per day. With Tourette's syndrome, supplementation with other amino acids and nutrients is extremely important. Research shows taurine helps reduce muscular spasms/rigidity in patients with muscular dystrophy.

A deficiency of taurine exists in patients with depression. If a depressed patient is environmentally sensitive, a taurine deficiency can compound chemical sensitivities, and decrease the body's ability to detoxify chemicals.

Taurine is necessary for the formation of one of the bile acids and for proper functioning of the gallbladder. Taurine, in doses of three to six grams daily, divided, increases bile production, which may prevent the formation of gallstones. The bile may be a route of

excretion of chemicals detoxified by the body. Taurine is sometimes called upon to help control inflammation or infection.

Taurine, or a modified taurine, may someday supersede syn-
thetic tranquilizers. Stress depletes the body of taurine. Whenever you experience more than usual amounts of stress, chronically, or if you have an illness, the need for taurine increases.
Chronic pain of any kind depletes the body of taurine. Often,
supplementation is necessary, as the need for taurine is greater
than what we can obtain from our diets. In over 300 amino acid
profiles done on patients at the Pain & Stress Center, nine out of
ten patients showed a deficiency of taurine. In most cases, one to
three grams of taurine supplementation was required daily.

Best food sources of taurine include meats, especially organ
meats, and fish. Supplementation is necessary, as the taurine need
becomes greater than what can be obtained from the diet, alone.

Usual dosage of taurine is 500 to 3,000 mg per day, preferably on an empty stomach. Women require more taurine than
men, since men have higher enzyme levels.

Our pets (domestic dogs and cats) need taurine, too. Most pets
are dependent upon their diet for taurine, but taurine is often absent
in commercially prepared foods. A deficiency of taurine causes
degeneration of the retina of the eye, often leading to blindness. To
ensure your pet obtains enough taurine, supplement the diet part of
the time with fresh meat (organ meats, liver, kidney, brains, heart)
or fish. These foods are the best sources of taurine for pets.

Threonine

Threonine is an essential amino acid, and is the precursor to
brain glycine. It is required for proper digestion and intestinal tract
function. Threonine breaks down into glucose, and into the amino
acids glycine and serine.

Deficiency of threonine suppresses the immune system. It has
been helpful in multiple sclerosis cases and in some patients with
agitated depression and mania.

Good food sources includes pork, turkey, wheat germ, and cottage and ricotta cheeses.

Tryptophan

Tryptophan is an essential amino acid, and must be obtained in the diet. It ultimately breaks down into serotonin, the calming neurotransmitter in the brain. Serotonin helps us feel calm, relaxed, and in control.

Tryptophan Pathway
Tryptophan → 5-HTP → Serotonin

Tryptophan is a precursor of serotonin. Serotonin is synthesized from tryptophan. Serotonin is a brain neurotransmitter, platelet-clotting factor, and neurohormone found in the organs throughout the body. Tryptophan is essential to maintaining the body's protein balance. When food that is protein deficient or lacking tryptophan is fed to growing or mature individuals, such foods fail to replace worn-out materials lost by the body during the organic activities of its cells, tissues, and organs. The amino acid tryptophan is exhausted by the vital activities of the body and, in turn, must be replaced to prevent atrophy of the body's structures.

One of the few substances capable of passing the blood-brain barrier, tryptophan plays a variety of important roles in mental activity. When tryptophan intake is deficient, especially during periods of stress, serotonin levels drop, causing depression, anxiety, insecurity, hyperactivity, insomnia, and pain. The body requires ample supplies of Vitamin B6 for the formation of tryptophan.

Tryptophan's role in behavior has been demonstrated by the number of mental functions it directly influences. Serotonin produces a relaxed, calm, secure, mellow, and morphine-like analgesic feeling. Only 1 to 2% of all serotonin in the body is found in the brain. Hyperactive children/adults have a low serotonin level. Aggression reflects one of the most widely recognized signs of reduced serotonin. Supplements containing tryptophan and Vitamin B6 can correct some of the biochemical disorders related to aggression.

Another significant finding in studies done with tryptophan demonstrated that low levels of serotonin could play a part in the development of depression. Combining tryptophan (1,000 mg) with tyrosine in doses of 3,000 mg per day, at bedtime, can mimic the effects of most antidepressants. Tryptophan is useful in unipolar depression or constant, low-grade depression with no highs or lows.

Both depression and pain can have profound effects on a person's ability to fall asleep. Difficulty in falling asleep can be caused by low serotonin levels. But tryptophan has been shown to effectively solve insomnia problems, reducing the time needed to fall asleep, and increasing the number of hours spent sleeping. The usual dosage is 500 to 1,000 mg, taken one hour prior to bedtime with a carbohydrate such as orange juice or fruit.

Because serotonin is a neurotransmitter, it is one of the most important chemicals to help control moods. Best of all, tryptophan is safe, and is a natural relaxant and tranquilizer of the central nervous system. The body has no difficulty in rapidly metabolizing and clearing it from the body. As an essential amino acid necessary for life, tryptophan is the sole precursor for serotonin. It does not simply pass through the gut into the brain, to become serotonin. It must compete with five other amino acids—tyrosine, phenylalanine, leucine, isoleucine, and valine—at the blood-brain barrier. In order to increase the amount of brain serotonin, the ratio of tryptophan must be elevated out of proportion to the competing amino acids. Metabolism and protein intake may alter this ratio.

About 90% of serum tryptophan is bound to albumin. Free fatty acids (serum) share the same albumin binding sites. Changing both the blood-sugar level and insulin may increase and decrease the proportion of free tryptophan that has access to the brain. In the total serum amino acid profile, the ratio of tryptophan to the nutrient amino acids has been elevated in each instance. Tyrosine has also been elevated in each instance. About 1% of the ingested tryptophan metabolizes to serotonin. About 90% of the tryptophan metabolizes through kynurenic acid to nicotinic acid.

The neurotransmitters directly depend on dietary tryptophan and other amino acids. Circadian rhythms effect the amino acid utilization in the nervous system. Circadian rhythm is a specific type of periodicity for the uptake and utilization of substances. This has recently been shown with use of tryptophan in the treatment of insomnia. When tryptophan is used during the day, it does not seem to induce sleep, only a calm, relaxed state; but when taken near bedtime, it seems to induce sleep, as shown in sleep studies done at several medical centers. This seems to indicate that tryptophan's uptake across the blood-brain barrier corresponds to the circadian rhythms of the sleep cycle. Its absorption and conversion in the brain to serotonin more effectively occurs during times when a person would normally sleep. This is why it is clinically suggested to administer tryptophan at bedtime, if used for treating sleep disorders. Conversely, tryptophan or tyrosine should be used during the day to treat certain forms of depression. Liquid homepathic serotonin used 3 to 4 times daily will elevate the serotonin level. Melatonin also elevates the serotonin level, and is effective for sleep problems. Melatonin is produced by the pineal gland in the brain, and is a neurohormone.

Two researchers in England compared the antidepressant effects of tryptophan and Tofranil. (Tofranil, or imipramine, is a drug commonly used for depression.) Both groups of patients with depression improved. The study revealed that tryptophan was just as effective as the laboratory-produced drug, and there were no side effects from the tryptophan. Conversely, the side effects for the Tofranil group included blurring of vision, dryness of the mouth, low blood pressure, urinary retention, heart palpitations, hepatitis, and seizures.

Tryptophan is obtained in the diet every day. Many rich natural forms of tryptophan include: bananas, green leafy vegetables, red meat, pork, turkey, dairy products, pineapple, avocados, eggs, soy, sesame and pumpkin seeds, and lentils. Large doses of tryptophan, when combined with niacinamide and Vitamin B6, can enhance the conversion of tryptophan to serotonin.

Currently, tryptophan is available only by prescription. It was removed for sale in 1989 because of a contaminated batch that caused EMS (eosinophilia-myalgia syndrome). The F.D.A. determined the cause was tryptophan and not the contaminated batch. It reclassified tryptophan as an unapproved experimental drug, and ordered recall of all products except where tryptophan occurred naturally. To date, tryptophan is still banned for sale in the U.S.

But within the last several years, 5-HTP, or 5-hydroxytryptophan, has become available. 5-HTP derives from griffonia seeds, a member of the legume or bean family. 5-HTP, about 10 times stronger than tryptophan, is one step closer to serotonin. Suggested dosage is 50 to 300 mg of 5-HTP, daily.

One study compared 5-HTP to Luvox, an antidepressant. Subjects with depression were given 100 mg of 5-HTP, three times daily, or 150 mg, of Luvox, three times daily. Evaluations were done at 2, 4, and 6 weeks. After 2 weeks, both groups reported a significant reduction in depression. By week 4, 15 of 36 5-HTP patients and 18 of 33 Luvox patients reported at least a 50% improvement in depression symptoms. Final assessment demonstrated the 5-HTP patients had the greatest improvement and the least amount of treatment failures. Another study involving endogenous depression (arising from within the individual, in all likelihood genetic) demonstrated marked improvement or cure in 69% of patients receiving 5-HTP.

Tyrosine

Tyrosine is the first breakdown product of phenylalanine, and is considered a nonessential amino acid because the body can make it from phenylalanine. Tyrosine is the *stress* amino acid.

Dr. Gelenberg, at Harvard Medical School, determined tyrosine is more effective than antidepressants for relief of depression. To rapidly increase the norepinephrine level, use tyrosine. Because it is one step closer to norepinephrine, you feel the effect more rapidly. Suggested amount of tyrosine is one 850 mg capsule of pharmaceutical grade tyrosine, three times daily. *Do not take tyrosine with MAO inhibitors or tricyclic antidepressants, or if you have schizophrenia.*

Researchers at Urije University, in the Netherlands, found supplementing with tyrosine enhanced memory and reduced blood pressure in healthy, young, military cadets. The cadets received either protein-rich drinks containing two grams tyrosine, or carbohydrate-rich drinks with equal calories. After six days, the supplemented cadets performed better on memory and tracking tests, and showed decreased systolic blood pressures. Researchers concluded that tyrosine supplementation might, under working conditions distinguished by psychosocial and physical stress, reduce the effects of stress and fatigue.

See the phenylalanine section for metabolism and specifics.

B.N.C.
Balanced Neurotransmitter Complex

The brain communicates through neurotransmitters, the chemical language of the brain. A balanced neurotransmitter complex contains the amino acids in a special blend that nourishes the brain. An unbalanced diet, anxiety, chronic pain, depression, and grief, plus other factors, can contribute to disturbances in amino acid metabolism. B.N.C. contains the special amino acid mix of phenylalanine, leucine, valine, histidine, arginine, lysine, isoleucine, alanine, glutamine, methionine, threonine, alpha-ketoglutaric acid, pyridoxal 5'phosphate (B6), and chromium picolinate. These 12 amino acids, plus activity agents, can be taken on a daily basis without fear of creating an amino acid imbalance. B.N.C. can be combined with other amino acids for a total orthomolecular approach. Research has shown substantial improvement in chronic fatigue patients using the B.N.C. complex, CoEnzyme Q10, Alpha KG, and Mag Link. B.N.C. should be taken on a daily basis to correct impairments in biochemistry that can either cause or complicate health conditions. Amino acids, because of their intimate involvement in metabolic regulation, prove very useful therapeutic agents that reverse biochemical impairments related to amino acid metabolism. B.N.C. has been instrumental in correcting mental and stress-related disturbances, food and chemical intolerances, learning disabilities, frequent headaches, fibromyalgia, chronic fatigue, mental and emotional disturbances, hyperactivity, and some neurological disorders. B.N.C. is available in capsule and powder forms.

Disorders Associated with Amino Acid Imbalances

- ADD/ADHD
- Alcoholism
- Ammonia toxicity
- Ataxia (defective muscular coordination)
- Behavioral disorders
- Cardiovascular disease
- Chemical intolerances
- Chronic fatigue
- Chronic gastrointestinal distress or bowel irregularity
- Depression
- Dermatitis (inflammation of the skin)
- Detoxification impairments
- Excessive inflammation
- Failure to thrive (infancy)
- Family history or early symptoms of degenerative disease
- Frequent headaches
- Frequent infections and persistent inflammatory responses
- Hyperlipidemias (high blood lipid levels)
- Hypertension (high blood pressure)
- Hypotonia (loss of muscle tone)
- Inflammatory disorders
- Impaired mental development
- Insomnia
- Intolerances (persistent) to foods and chemicals
- Mental disperception
- Mental retardation
- Myopathies (muscular diseases)
- Neurological disorders
- Neural tube defects (birth defects)
- Ocular disorders (eye)
- Osteoporosis
- Oxidative stress
- Poor immunity
- Poor wound healing
- Rheumatoid arthritis
- Seizures
- Short stature or chronically underweight, growth failure (children)
- Weak skin and nails

Source: *Diagnostic Value of Amino Acid Analysis*, Great Smokies Diagnostic Laboratory,

Amino Acid Cofactors

B6

Pyridoxine

Due to its function in the body, B6 is one of the most important vitamins the body needs. B6 transforms to pyridoxal 5'phosphate, or P5'P. P5'P is a coenzyme that activates enzymes and enzyme systems. Our bodies could not function without enzymes because they trigger *every* chemical reaction within the body. One hundred eighteen enzymes and nineteen of the twenty amino acids rely on Vitamin B6. B6 serves as a catalyst for the enzymes in the body, and without it we could not digest amino acids (proteins), carbohydrates, and fats. B6 is necessary for life. B6 and magnesium are necessary cofactors for proper brain function.

At Tufts University a study by the U.S. Department of Agriculture Human Nutrition Research Center on Aging, revealed the elderly need at least 3 milligrams of Vitamin B6, daily. B6 should not be taken in dosages greater than 300 mg, per day. Daily ingestion of over 300 mg of B6 can cause irreversible neurotoxicity. Neurotoxicity involves dosages of B6 too high or toxic to the nerves in the dorsal root ganglia (spinal cord) and to sensory nerves in the feet and legs. Dr. Karl Folkers, of Clayton Foundation, University of Texas, determined daily dosages of 50 to 300 milligrams of B6 to be safe for adults over seventeen years, including pregnant women, and patients with diabetes, heart disease, or

---

U.S. Recommended Daily Allowance (USRDAs) for B6

0.3 milligrams, for infants six to eleven months old;

1 milligram, for children nine to thirteen years of age;

1.5 milligrams, for females fourteen to eighteen years of age;

1.7 milligrams, for males fourteen to eighteen years of age;

2.2 milligrams, for pregnant women;

2 milligrams, for adult males.

Signs and Symptoms of Vitamin B6 Deficiency in the Human Body

The following signs and symptoms may indicate a Vitamin B6 deficiency.

- Paresthesia (pins-and-needles numbness and tingling in distal parts of the hands or feet) in the hands or feet
- Impaired sensation in the fingers
- Impaired flexion of the finger joints
- Fluctuating edema in the hands
- Morning stiffness in the fingers
- Pain in the hands
- Impaired coordination of the fingers
- Weakness of pinch (the pressure point between the thumb and index finger)
- Increased tendency to drop objects
- Tenderness over the carpal tunnel with Tinel's sign (a tingling sensation radiating out into the hand and accompanied by pain at the wrist) and Phalen's sign (Paresthesia in the fingers that becomes worse when the median nerve is squeezed between the ligament and tendons while the wrist is held flexed for thirty to sixty seconds.)
- Pain in the shoulders
- Pain upon movement of the thumb knuckle (metacarpophalangeal joint)
- Pain in the elbows
- Sleep paralysis (the temporary inability to lift the arm or hand upon awakening during the night)
- Edema from steroid-hormone therapy (a puffy swelling in the tissues of the face, hands, feet, or legs when steroid hormones, particularly when taking large doses of cortisone or female hormones such as estrogen)
- Macular edema (an abnormal collection of fluid and fatty substances that have leaked from tiny arteries near the central portion of the retina of the eye, resulting in disturbed central vision)

If you notice any of these signs and symptoms, contact your physician. You may find Vitamin-B6 therapy extremely helpful. Source: *Vitamin B6 Therapy*, by John M. Ellis, M.D. and Jean Pamplin; p. 43.

carpal tunnel syndrome. B6 may improve or prevent acne, alcoholism, asthma, heart disease, diabetes, hyperactivity, PMS, repetitive stress injury, and pregnancy/toxemia.

The body requires B6 and four minerals, especially if you have diabetes or any diabetic complications. The four minerals comprise chromium, magnesium, zinc, and potassium. Studies demonstrate that B6 slows the development of diabetic complications such as diabetic retinopathy, kidney problems, or heart disease. Evidence suggests that diabetics who have taken 100 to 300 mg, daily, for several years, are more likely to survive a heart attack and live longer than diabetics not supplementing with B6.

B6 functions in the liver, brain, blood, muscles, cartilage, bone, hormones, arteries, etc., are still under investigation by scientists. Elevated homocysteine levels in the blood contribute to changes in arteries and the development of heart disease. At New York University Medical Center, studies proved that high levels of homocysteine and low levels of B6 contribute to severe calcification in the aortas of patients with advanced atherosclerosis. Calcified deposits promote blockage of arteries. B6 is readily destroyed with baking or other cooking. Heat destroys B6. You should take B6 as a time-released form (150 mg) that releases over eight to nine hours, or take pyridoxal-5-phosphate (P5'P), the biological form of B6.

Timed Release Rodex B6

Supplementation with timed-released B6 disperses B6 over a period of 8 to 9 hours. This timed-release B6 helps prevent neurotoxicity which can occur in doses greater than 500 mg over a prolonged period of time.

P5'P or Pyridoxal 5'Phosphate
Active B6

Pyridoxal 5' Phosphate, or P5'P, the biological (active) form of B6 is necessary for the utilization of all amino acids, proteins, fats, and carbohydrates. If P5'P is not present, increased excretion of most amino acids occurs as well as increased formation of abnormal amino acid metabolites.

Unlike B6 there is no fear of toxicity with P5'P, even in children. Reaction to MSG may indicates a deficiency of P5'P or Vitamin B6. Reactions to MSG may effectively be prevented with supplementation of B6 or P5'P.

Magnesium

Magnesium is an essential cofactor in over 300 enzyme reactions in the body. Many Americans are deficient in magnesium, and do not get enough from their diets. Magnesium and B6, or P5'P, must be present or the body cannot assimilate and properly use amino acids.

Magnesium is known as the stress mineral. As an essential cofactor in over 300 enzyme reactions that occur in the body, magnesium is necessary for energy production and DNA replication, the basis of all life. Currently, doctors emphasize calcium supplements for the prevention and treatment of osteoporosis. While trying to get sufficient quantities of calcium, the majority of people pay little attention to their intake of magnesium. But magnesium plays an important role in bone health.

Magnesium, like calcium, helps promote healthy bones and teeth, decreases high blood pressure, and maintains muscle health. Like calcium, magnesium is distributed throughout the body. Most magnesium is found in the bones, which store this essential mineral. A profound difference exists between calcium and magnesium at the cellular levels. Calcium concentrates outside the cell, while magnesium finds its way inside all body cells. The body needs both minerals to maintain electrical potential across the cell membranes, or simply, they assist the transmission of nerve impulses. *Just as calcium is required for muscle contraction, magnesium is essential for muscle relaxation.* Recent research demonstrates that humans require magnesium in a balance of 2 parts magnesium to 1 part calcium.

Until the age of 35, bone mass can increase. Bone loss occurs due to an imbalance of the modeling process, and bones begin to lose both their mineral and their gelatinous matrix. Menopause, or the change of life for a woman, usually precipitates a bone crisis. During the change-of-life years, rapid declines in bone mass occur making women more susceptible to bone fractures. Fewer fractures occur in women supplementing with magnesium and calcium than in women supplementing with only calcium. If you increase your calcium intake, it is vitally important that you also increase your intake of magnesium.

More than fifty percent of doctor visits are for fatigue. Modern medicine offers little for this problem. If you provide your body all the nutrients it needs for energy production, your fatigue will often decrease. Magnesium proves essential for energy production in the cells. Magnesium helps relieve Chronic Fatigue Syndrome (CFS). Studies show that red-blood-cell magnesium levels measure considerably lower in CFS patients than in normal patients.

Magnesium deficiency causes release of more histamine. Histamine releases whenever you react to an allergen that triggers an allergic reaction to a food, chemical, or environmental factor. Low levels of magnesium contribute to kidney-stone formation. Daily supplementation with magnesium and B6 promotes removal and prevents reformation of kidney stones. A four-year study of fifty-five patients demonstrated that ingesting 500 mg of magnesium, daily, reduced by ninety percent the reformation of kidney stones. The control group that did not supplement with magnesium experienced a reoccurrence rate of 41%. Magnesium deficiency leads to neuromuscular malfunctions such as tremors, convulsions, high excitability, behavior disorders, neuromuscular pain, and depression. Magnesium acts as a muscle relaxant, reducing the spasms in PMS, menstrual cramps, fibromyalgia, trigger points, muscle cramps, or any other painful condition. Supplementing with magnesium chloride produced the best results.

Supplementing with magnesium is safe. Excessive magnesium occurs only in people with kidney problems or impaired kidney function. Magnesium can cause loose stools, or diarrhea, in some people. If this occurs, divide the dosage of magnesium into three to six times a day and night, or try a different form of magnesium. The best-tolerated form of magnesium is a magnesium chloride tablet, such as Mag Link.

The majority of healthcare practitioners do not realize that increasing intakes of refined carbohydrates and processed foods

Magnesium/Amino Acid Connection

Symptoms of Magnesium *Deficiency*

- Anxiety
- Panic attacks
- Mitral valve prolapse
- Hypertension
- Chronic pain
- Back and neck pain
- Muscle spasms
- Migraines
- Fibromyalgia
- Spastic symptoms
- Chronic bronchitis, emphysema
- Vertigo (dizziness)
- Confusion
- Depression
- Psychosis
- Noise sensitivity
- Ringing in the ears
- Irritable-bowel syndrome
- Cardiovascular disease
- Cardiac arrhythmias
- Atherosclerosis/Intermittent claudication
- Raynaud's disease (cold hands and feet)
- TIA's (Transient Ischemic Attacks-strokes)
- Constipation
- Fatigue
- Diabetes
- Hypoglycemia
- Asthma
- Seizures
- Kidney stones
- Premenstrual syndrome
- Menstrual cramps
- Osteoporosis

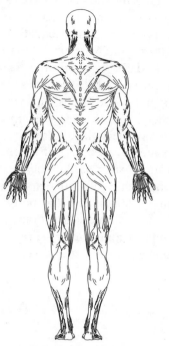

You have 657 muscles that need magnesium every second of every day. Magnesium is a cofactor for all amino acids.

For maximum benefit, add some magnesium in the form of magnesium chloride such as Mag Link. Try two tablets, twice to three times daily. If loose stools or diarrhea occur, decrease by one tablet or try increasing amount of time between doses. You should begin to feel a decrease in symptoms.

Warning: People with renal or kidney failure should not take magnesium without medical supervision.

For detailed information on magnesium-deficiency symptoms, read *The Anxiety Epidemic* by Dr. Sahley.

increase the body's requirement for magnesium. If magnesium intake has not kept pace, subliminal deficiency occurs. Most Americans do not get enough magnesium and other vital nutrients. The recommended daily value (RDV) for magnesium is 400 mg. The typical American diet provides between 200–300 mg, daily. Dr. Mildred Seelig, a nationally recognized magnesium specialist, estimates deficiencies in over 80 percent of the population. Reevaluate your diet and current health status, and add the needed magnesium to your supplement program. Ingestion of alcohol, soft drinks, and processed foods—all high in phosphates—cause loss of magnesium via the kidney. Certain medications such as diuretics, asthma medications such as theophylline, being over 40 years of age, and diabetes increase the loss of magnesium from the body. Rich food sources of magnesium include whole-wheat flour, nuts—almonds, brazils, cashews, peanuts, peanut butter—green leafy vegetables, soybeans, lentils, boiled shrimp, snails, yeast, brown rice, and dried peas.

Alpha KG

Alpha KG and citric acid are elements of the Krebs cycle (TCA cycle), the chemical engine that generates energy for every cell of the body. Alpha KG works with B6 and magnesium to metabolize amino acids, thus enabling the body to convert amino acids into other substances it needs. Proper brain neurotransmitter production requires optimal amino acid metabolism. Alpha KG + is a combination formula intended to address metabolic deficiencies seen in human plasma amino acid analyses. Alpha KG contains Alpha-Ketoglutaric acid, potassium and magnesium citrates and aspartates, B6, and Vitamin C (Ascorbyl Palmitate).

The components of Alpha KG + work at various sites of metabolic deficiencies. When given orally, Alpha KG + drives the Krebs cycle forward that greatly enhances cellular energy, thus decreasing fatigue and increasing stamina. Magnesium and potassium aspartates indirectly contribute to increased energy. In double-blind clinical trials, magnesium and potassium aspartates proved effective for the treatment of chronic fatigue.

Important Note

This section of the book divides into generalized categories by condition. Each condition includes suggested nutritional support with the most important amino acids, or combinations of amino acids (specific formulas that work), for that particular condition. To comprehensively cover certain conditions, other vitamins, herbs, or nutrients are included in this section.

Note: You do not need to take all of the amino acids or nutrients listed.

Pick the aminos that apply to your symptoms, or start with a few items, and see how you feel. You can always add another amino acid or nutrient, later. If you slowly add nutrients, you will know what is helping and what is not.

Example 1. If you use the Brain Link Complex formulation that contains glutamine, you do not necessarily need to add more glutamine to your diet.

Example 2. If you have a problem with memory, start with BNC and glutamine; then if needed, add ginkgo or huperzine.

If you have questions regarding the specific supplements listed, call 1-800-669-2256.

Amino Acids in Therapy

Addiction (Alcohol)

Alcoholism is a disease of chemical dependency. It is addictive, abusive, and eventually becomes destructive. Alcoholism ranks with stress, mental illness, and heart disease as one of the major problems in the U.S. Alcoholism develops from a combination of factors—psychological, physiological, genetic, and environmental. Presently, records show alcohol is the most abused drug in the U.S., and the problem is on the increase, especially among teenagers.

Researchers have established multiple nutrient deficiencies in those craving alcohol. Many are predisposed to alcoholism because of genetics. Those who have alcoholic parents or grandparents will have the same brain deficiencies which can lead to addictive behavior.

Dr. Roger Williams and his colleagues at the Clayton Foundation for Research at the University of Texas, established the vital research concerning the amino acid L-glutamine. Those craving alcohol have a definite glutamine deficiency. Dr. Williams and his associates observed that glutamine protects individuals against the poisonous effects of alcohol, and that it stopped the craving for alcohol. They studied all the properties of glutamine and GABA, and found those who had addictive behaviors had deficiencies.

Glutamine and GABA will decrease the craving for alcohol. Pure glutamine is tasteless, and can be mixed with food, water, or taken in capsule form. One alcoholic who was part of the study stopped drinking after he was given 3,000 mg of glutamine, daily, along with other necessary nutrients. Several studies demonstrated glutamine effectively reduces the craving for sweets. The same appetite center in the brain and hypothalamus protects against alcohol craving. Glutamine is the third most abundant amino acid in the blood and brain. Glutamine provides a major alternative fuel source when blood-sugar levels are low. Amino acids create the needed neurotransmitters to enhance the brain chemistry. A strong nutritional program is of utmost importance for the control of alcoholism and addictive behaviors.

For more information about addiction, especially prescribed addiction, read our book entitled, *Breaking Your Prescribed Addiction.*

Suggested Nutritional Support

Glutamine powder or caps – 1,000 to 4,000 mg per day, divided.

Rodex B6 (timed release) – 1 (150 mg) capsule per day.

B Complex – 1 capsule per day.

Mag Link – 4 to 6 per day, divided. Take to bowel tolerance then decrease by 1.

Ester C – 2,000 to 3,000 mg daily, divided.

Tyrosine 850* – 1 (850 mg) twice per day for depression.

Mood Sync** – 1 or 2 capsules, twice to three times daily for depression.

Anxiety Control 24 – 2 twice to three times per day, as needed, for stress and anxiety.

T-L Vite (multivitamin) – 1 capsule with breakfast

Or Use **Brain Link** – 2 scoops in the morning, depending on weight; if over 200 pounds, use 3 scoops.

DLPA* 750 mg – two, twice daily. (Do not use if you are taking MAO inhibitor or tricyclic antidepressants).

Cal, Mag, Zinc – 4 per day, at bedtime.

Liquid Serotonin – 10 to 12 drops, four times per day.

5-HTP** – 1 to 2 capsule (50 mg) an hour before bedtime, with juice.

* Tyrosine, Phenylalanine, or DLPA should not be taken by pregnant or lactating women, those with PKU, if you are taking MAO inhibitors or tricyclic antidepressants, or if you have had a malignant melanoma.

** Do not use if you are taking any SSRI medications.

The mind suffers. . . the body cries . . . the brain starves . . .

Adult A.D.D. / Hyperactivity

Recently, there has been an increase in the number of adults who feel they have ADD or ADHD, major problems they describe include their inability to concentrate, complete tasks, or stay focused. Many of them have turned to the powerful drug, Ritalin. Stimulant drugs such as Ritalin impair brain function and have no beneficial effect on the brain. According to Peter Breggin, M.D., in his book, *Talking Back to Ritalin,* Ritalin can either shrink or limit the growth of some areas of the brain, just as many psychiatric drugs can cause brain dysfunction and damage.

There are 16 adverse reactions listed in the PDR (*Physicians' Desk Reference*) for Ritalin. The most common adverse reactions are nervousness and insomnia. Other reactions include skin rashes, fever, anorexia, dizziness, palpitations, headaches, dyskinesia, drowsiness, blood pressure and pulse changes, pulse >100, angina, cardiac arrhythmias (heart rhythm disturbances), abdominal pain, and weight loss. Given this information, there should be no question about your decision.

There is no such thing as a Ritalin deficiency! There are many reasons why as we age our memory might not be what we feel it should be, but Ritalin is *not* the answer. Your brain cannot be deficient of Ritalin. If you cannot concentrate or stay focused, you need neurotransmitters. The following nutritional support program will help you nourish your brain so you feel better and think more clearly.

Suggested Nutritional Support

Brain Link Complex – 2 scoops in the morning, depending on weight; if over 200 pounds, 3 scoops.

Glutamine – 500 mg capsule, twice daily.

Mood Sync* – 1 capsule in the morning, afternoon, and evening.

Mag Link – 1 tablet, three times per day.

Ginkgo Biloba – 40 mg capsule, twice daily.

5-HTP* – 1 capsule, 30 minutes prior to bedtime.

Huperzine – 50 mcg capsule in the morning and in the evening.

* Do not use if you are taking any SSRI, tricyclic or MAO inhibitor medications.

Huperzine derives from purified Chinese club moss and is a premier brain nutrient. Clinical studies confirm Huperzine enhances memory, and can be used by anyone twelve years of age or older. *Do not use if you are a pregnant or lactating woman, or if you have heart or pulmonary problems.*

Phosphatidylserine – 1 to 3 capsules daily, divided. Phosphatidylserine (PS) is a phospholipid that is a component of brain cell membranes. Clinical studies demonstrate PS helps improve cognitive functions that decline with age including memory, learning, concentration, and vocabulary skills. Daily supplementation of PS provides more alertness and protects you against brain strain.

Special Note: If your symptoms become acute after you eat certain foods, your problems could be related to food allergies. Millions of children and adults are diagnosed with ADD or ADHD when their problem is really food allergy related. For detailed information regarding ADD and ADHD, read my book, *Control Hyperactivity/ A.D.D. Naturally.* It is available at your health food store or through the Pain & Stress Center at 1-800-669-2256.

Allergies / Sinus Problems

Allergies are the cause of sinus congestion and problems in about 90% of sinus cases. If you experience constant congestion and pressure, allergies could be the problem. Explore the possibility of chemical allergens as well as airborne. Food sensitivities/ allergies can also cause congestion, stuffiness, headache, palpitations, upset stomach, fatigue, etc. If you eliminate or rotate the foods that contribute to your sinus problems, you help your body detoxify. Rotate your foods so you do not eat a particular food/ food group any more frequently than every four to five days. For example, if you eat milk or milk products on Sunday, you would not eat any milk product until Thursday or Friday. The time interval allows your body to recover from the exposure to the food you are sensitive to. So you feel better, have more energy, and have less problems with your allergies and sinuses.

Do not get hooked on nasal decongestant sprays such as Duration. Nasal decongestants have a rebound effect requiring you to use them repeatedly. Instead use some saline (salt water) or MSM crystals dissolved in distilled water to rinse your nose. Then use the homeopathic sprays.

Suggested Nutritional Support

NAC (N-Acetyl-Cysteine) – 1 600 mg capsule, twice to three times per day.

P5'P – 100 mg, morning and evening.

Tyrosine (500 mg) – 1 capsule in morning and 1 in evening. Do not use if you are taking MAO inhibitors, tricyclic antidepressants, or if you have had a malignant melanoma.

Vitamin C (Ester C) – 2,000 mg, three times per day.

Mag Link – 4 to 6 tablets per day, divided. Magnesium helps prevent release of histamine. If diarrhea or loose stools occur, take tablets more divided or decrease dosage by 1.

Pycnogenol – 300 mg per day. Pycnogenol, or OPC, has great antioxidant value due to its free radical scavenging ability.

BHI Sinus (homeopathic) – 1 tablet every 15 minutes until improvement; then decrease to once every hour; then 1 tablet, four times per day.

BHI Allergy (homeopathic) – 1 tablet every 15 minutes until improvement; then decrease to once every hour; then 1 tablet, four times daily for allergic symptoms.

BHI Headache (homeopathic) – For sinus headache, use 1 tablet every 15 minutes until relief; then decrease to once every hour; then 1 tablet, four times per day.

MSM wash – Mix 1500 mg MSM crystals in 1½ ounces of distilled water. Using a bulb syringe, tilt your head to side and rinse each sinus.

Euphorbium Nasal Spray – Use as needed for nasal congestion. Euphorbium helps normalize nasal tissues, and does not have a rebound effect.

Sinus & Allergy Nasal Spray (SAS) – 1 or 2 sprays into each nostril every four hours, or as needed. SAS is a natural homeopathic medicine without fear of histamine rebound. SAS provides temporary relief for symptoms associated with inflamed nasal passages such as sinus pressure and headache, congestion, runny nose, dry nasal passages, and sneezing. Use SAS year round for sinus and allergies due to respiratory allergies to pollen, animals, molds, yeast, or dust.

Oil of Oregano – Use 6 drops in fruit juice for chronic congestion. Make sure the oregano is *wild oregano*. In addition, use Oregano capsules; 2 capsules, three times per day, for chronic allergies and sinusitis.

Anti-Aging

Only you have the potential to change the way you live and age. Once you reach age 40, you hold the key to your productivity, your life-style, and the quality of your life. What is aging? Aging is breathing. Breathing oxygen produces free radicals that attack our cells! In effect, the very air you breathe in order to live, simultaneously causes you to age by rusting your body. In your teens and twenties, your cells were able to repair the damage caused by constant free radicals; but with age, oxygen attacks the body's mechanisms that replace and repair. With age, you become susceptible to damage from free radicals to your cell metabolism and your DNA. If you are over the age of 40, the damaging free-radical process is now in place.

Once in the body, free radicals attack cell components and damage cells and tissues in the body. This free-radical-induced damage alters the cell membrane structure and function. The membrane is no longer able to transport nutrients, oxygen, and water into the cell, and can no longer regulate the removal of waste products.

Free radicals also damage the cell's mitochondria, resulting in limited or halted production of energy for all cell processes. Free-radical damage to enzymes and other proteins limits the body's building of tissues and causes accumulation of protein fragments. Both these conditions are recognized in premature aging of tissues. Finally, a cell cannot reproduce normally when free radicals alter the genetic code. Last resort: the cell dies, or the cell mutates to a cancerous cell.

Free radicals in the body are unavoidable. They form as a result of normal metabolic processes—during the formation of prostaglandins, or from normal intracellular oxygen metabolism. Free radicals are consumed in some foods, inhaled from air pollution and tobacco smoke, and generated in the environment from radiation and herbicides.

Fortunately, your body can use anti-free-radicals comprising antioxidants such as Vitamins C and E, beta-carotene, CoEnzyme Q10, NAC (N-Acetyl Cysteine), selenium, and glutathione. This powerful free-radical combination is available in one capsule: the

Deluxe Scavenger. The recommended dose is 3 capsules, daily. The Deluxe Scavengers protect the cells from free-radical damage.

As the aging process progresses, other physiological changes take place, including increased fat levels and decreased muscle mass. Additionally, you have decreased bone mass, decreased water intake and content, and increased fatigue. No two people age the same, so the exact point at which decline begins is different for everyone. The majority of gerontologists agree that 50 seems to be the magic number.

The key to controlling the aging process is to assist the brain and body to recreate homeostasis of youth. How do you do this? By supplying needed nutrients such as growth hormone, the connecting link between the brain and body. Scientists have found that amino acids will induce growth hormone secretion. The amino acid, glutamine, is most used by the body during times of stress, anxiety, depression, grief, and chronic pain. Your immune system and gut live on glutamine. If your body does not produce enough glutamine, you will experience memory and focus problems, muscle loss, as well as immune dysfunction. Your gut will atrophy, keeping valuable nutrients from being absorbed.

According to Dr. Ronald Klatz, President of the Academy of Anti-Aging Medicine, and author of *Grow Young with HGH,* glutamine is an effective growth hormone releaser that crosses

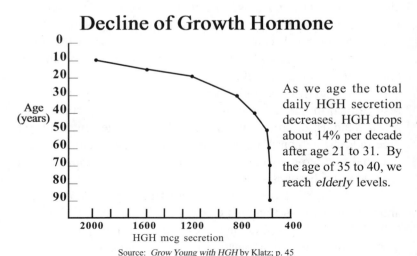

Decline of Growth Hormone

Age (years)

As we age the total daily HGH secretion decreases. HGH drops about 14% per decade after age 21 to 31. By the age of 35 to 40, we reach *elderly* levels.

HGH mcg secretion

Source: *Grow Young with HGH* by Klatz; p. 45

the blood-brain barrier where it increases energy and mental alertness. People with low glutamine levels have higher rates of arthritis, diabetes, and heart disease; those with high glutamine levels feel and perform much better. The recommended dose is 2 grams of glutamine powder at bedtime and an additional gram may be used in the morning for a jump-start. Glutamine is an inhibitory neurotransmitter vital in smooth brain function.

DHEA, a neurohormone produced primarily by the adrenal cortex, is the most abundant steroid hormone in humans. In his book, *DHEA, The Youth Hormone*, C. Norman Shealy, M.D., reports DHEA deficiencies in all patients with major diseases, including those with obesity, diabetes, high blood pressure, cancer, various immune deficiencies, coronary artery disease, and autoimmune disorders. Chronic stress syndrome uses available DHEA in the brain in concentrations equal to those in the adrenal cortex. Dr. Shealy's research "established the most important metabolic effects of DHEA: it stabilizes glucose, regulates all other hormones, decreases cholesterol, acts as a precursor to estrogen and testosterone, assists homeostasis due to chronic stress, enhances immune function, maintains youth and health, and stabilizes weight." DHEA should not be used until after the age of 40, unless blood tests verify your DHEA level to be low. The recommended dosage is to start with 25 mg, upon awakening in the morning; if you are over the age of 50 or weigh over 200 pounds, start with 50 mg. The best way to establish your needs is to have your blood tested for DHEA sulfate level. This will tell you exactly what your body needs. Most major labs can do this test.

Other Anti-Aging Nutritional Support

CoEnzyme Q10 – 30 to 150 mg, per day. CoEnzyme Q10 helps support the immune system, heart, and helps control the flow of oxygen within the cells.

Vitamin C (Ester C) – 2,000 to 3,000 mg, divided. Ester C is an antioxidant and helps support your immune system.

Vitamin E – 800 I.U., per day. Vitamin E is an antioxidant that helps retard aging and helps protect the heart and blood vessels.

Huperzine A – 1 (50 mcg) capsule in the morning, for memory and mind enhancement. Huperzine derives from purified Chinese club moss. Clinical studies confirm Huperzine enhances memory. Huperzine was featured in the *Journal of American Medical Association* (JAMA), and is recommended by neurologists. *Do not use Huperzine if you are a pregnant or lactating woman, or if you have heart or pulmonary problems.*

Brain Link Complex – 2 to 3 scoops, twice daily.

Neuromins – 1 to 2 (500 mg) capsules, in the morning and evening. More than 60% of the human brain is composed of fat, especially an omega-3 fatty acid called decosahexaenoic acid (DHA). DHA is needed for optimal signal transmissions in the brain, nervous system, and the eye, and is essential in the diet. Foods such as fish and egg yolks are rich sources of DHA.

Flax – 1 heaping teaspoon, twice daily, dissolved in juice or sprinkled over a food such as salad. Fortified flax is a rich source of omega 3, plus it provides fiber to help alleviate constipation and keep your intestines healthy.

Digestive enzymes (such as Super Digestaway and/or Pancreatin) – 1 capsule with each meal. As we age, we do not replace the enzymes lost with eating, so our enzyme levels decrease in the body.

Mag Link – 1 to 2 tablets, three to four times daily. Mag Link provides magnesium chloride, the same form of magnesium present in the body, so it is readily absorbed and tolerated.

Cal, Mag, Zinc – 4 capsules, at bedtime.

Melatonin – 1 (3 mg) capsule, 30 minutes to an hour prior to bedtime. Use melatonin only if you are over 30 years of age. Melatonin helps promote sleep and is a powerful antioxidant.

Pregnenolone – 10 to 50 mg daily, upon awakening in the morning. Pregnenolone is a direct precursor to DHEA and progesterone, and serves as the building block for all other steroid hormones. When the pregnenolone level drops, usually when you reach the age of 30, it negatively affects your mental function, memory, mood, and energy levels.

NAC (N-Acetyl Cysteine) – 1 capsule, twice daily. NAC is a precursor to glutathione, an antioxidant, and natural decongestant. Glutathione protects the body against natural and man-made oxidants.

Calm Colon – for IBS problems. See IBS section.

Brain Boosters
Memory and Concentration

The brain is the busiest, yet the most undernourished organ in the body. The brain is the master controller, the programmer for every movement, mood, breath, heartbeat, thought, even for body temperature and hormone balance. Our brain uses 20% of the body's total energy supply, so energy must be supplied on a constant basis in the form of nutrition and nutrients. Oxygen and glucose are in constant demand as fuel by the brain. The brain uses 25% of the body's total oxygen intake. Blood carries these nutrients to the brain at a rate of 1½ pints per minute. The brain uses oxygen and glucose first, then protein, fat, amino acids, vitamins, and minerals. Research has demonstrated that poor nutrition at any time in our life can permanently alter brain development.

Your state of nutrition equals the state of your brain's health and functioning. How your brain functions depends on how you nourish your mind and body, especially in today's stressful world. Stress and anxiety severely deter proper brain function. The quality of brain function depends on neurotransmitters, the chemical language of the brain. Neurotransmitters carry impulses from one neuron to another, as from one cell to another cell, such as a muscle cell. Neurotransmitters can either be inhibitory or excitatory. The balance determines whether motor neurons fire. If stress, anxiety, depression, or chronic pain cause major deficiencies, irregular firing can occur. Irregular firing of motor neurons sends mixed messages to the brain and can cause you to display maladaptive behavior.

Since 1975, scientists have identified more than fifty neurotransmitters, but the communications conducted between brain cells use only approximately ten major neurotransmitters. The best-known neurotransmitters are serotonin, epinephrine, norepinephrine, and acetylcholine. Serotonin comes from the precursor amino acid tryptophan, or 5-HTP. Epinephrine synthesizes from the amino acid phenylalanine, or tyrosine. Acetylcholine metabolizes from the B complex substance known as choline.

The following nutrients are important for proper brain function.

BNC (Balanced Neurotransmitter Complex®) helps maintain a balance of amino acids in the brain. BNC contains a balance of the amino acids phenylalanine, leucine, valine, histidine, arginine, lysine, isoleucine, alanine, glutamine, methionine, and threonine. Alpha-ketoglutaric acid, Pyridoxal 5 phosphate (B6), and Chromium Picolinate act as activating agents. Either children or adults can use this formula.

Glutamine was established as the memory and concentration amino acid by University of Texas premier researcher Dr. Roger Williams. Glutamine is found in the nerves of the hippocampus—the memory center of the brain, in the cranial nerves, and in numerous receptors throughout the brain and body. As the third-most abundant amino acid in the blood and brain, glutamine helps the brain dispose of waste ammonia, a protein breakdown by-product. Glutamine provides a major alternative fuel source for the brain with low blood-sugar levels. Ginkgo Biloba, a brain-booster herb, has an excellent track record for enhancing memory and concentration. Ginkgo increases blood flow to the head, and improves mental functioning and the ability to focus for longer periods of time. Senior citizens report excellent results combining Ginkgo and Glutamine.

Huperzine serrata, or Chinese club moss, comes from the mountains of China. This herb has been used for centuries to improve memory, focus, and concentration, and to help alleviate memory problems among the elderly. Research data indicates an estimated 100,000 people have been successfully treated. Huperzine is safe and effective as reported in the *Journal of the American Medical Association.* Huperzine, a natural, potent, and selective cholinesterase inhibitor proves superior to other acetyl-cholinesterase inhibitors. Scientific research demonstrates multiple therapeutic benefits of Huperzine use in the following areas: learning and memory retention, improved focus and concentration, treatment of cognitive and memory impairment, and improved nerve transmission signals to muscles. Huperzine A has been very effective for those suffering from Alzheimer's disease. Alzheimer's patients go through a progressive loss of neuron groups that inhibits communication in the brain and causes destruction of the cerebral cortex, the outer tissue of the brain. A major characteristic of Alzheimer's and progressive loss of mental cognitive function is oxidative stress that increases the rate at which the disease progresses. *If you have a problem with heart or pulmonary disease, or if you are pregnant or lactating, you should not use Huperzine.*

Oxidative stress results from free-radical damage. Brain cells are very susceptible to oxidative stress. To protect the brain from oxidative stress, you must take antioxidants on a daily basis. The Deluxe Scavengers formula contains the antioxidants CoQ10, Beta-Carotene, Vitamin C, Selenium, Glutathione, NAC, and B6, all in one capsule.

Minerals prove vital to brain function, and magnesium, as well as acting as a major cofactor for all amino acids, ensures smooth muscle function. You have 657 muscles in your body that require magnesium every second of every day. The best source of magnesium is Mag Link, magnesium chloride, the same form of magnesium that naturally occurs in your cells.

Phosphatidylserine (PS) revitalizes cognitive functions that decline with age—memory, learning, concentration, even vocabulary skills. Extremely well documented, PS has been researched in more than 60 human clinical studies over a period of more than 20 years, in both North America and Europe. Seventeen double-blind, controlled, clinical trials prove, beyond doubt, the considerable worth of PS as a dietary supplement. These consistently positive clinical findings, backed by more than 2,800 scientific research papers, prove that PS safely and effectively supports memory, learning, concentration, word recall, and a wide range of other cognitive brain functions.

Besides benefiting cognition, PS benefits other brain activities, like coping with stress, fighting depression, and maintaining daily hormone rhythms. In young, healthy men, PS lowered the production of stress hormones linked to strenuous exercise, and eased stress-related mood symptoms in the elderly. Phosphatidylserine enriches all our brain cells, which helps them produce and release the natural chemical transmitters that make the brain work.

But, while drugs can be used to raise or lower the levels of single chemical transmitters, PS influences many major transmitter systems to produce an overall harmonizing influence on the brain.

Phosphatidylserine also helps the brain process energy. The brain requires a lot of energy to carry out its function. The membranes of the mitochondria—the energy powerhouses of the nerve cells—carry out the vast majority of the cell energy functions. PS gets into these membranes, alongside Coenzyme Q10 and Vitamin E, improving energy efficiency.

For those who require all their vitamins, minerals, and amino acids in one complex, Brain Link, a complete neurotransmitter complex, supplies the body and brain with all the needed nutrients. Brain Link proves excellent for children, or adults, and can be mixed with any fruit juice. Brain Link is especially effective for those who have absorption problems and require a faster breakdown of nutrients.

Pregnenolone, the superhormone for your brain, enhances memory, improves concentration, and fights mental fatigue. Pregnenolone is one key to keeping your brain functioning at peak capacity even into your 80s. Some scientists believe it is the most-potent memory enhancer of all time. Pregnenolone is produced in the brain and in the adrenal cortex, the gland that sits above the kidneys. Pregnenolone production declines with age. By the time you reach 75 you produce 60% less pregnenolone than you did in your 30s. Superhormones, like pregnenolone, are similar to neurotransmitters. Located in the brain, they have a profound impact on mental function. Pregnenolone works with the amino acid GABA to enhance brain function. Clinical studies demonstrate that those with low levels of pregnenolone have clinical depression, as well as memory and concentration problems.

The brain is a super computer—but a computer must have constant nourishment to continue to produce the data we need, from childhood to our golden years.

Nutritional Support

BNC – 1 or 2 capsules in the morning. BNC provides needed neurotransmitters to improve memory and concentration. If you require additional GABA, you may prefer to use the BNC + GABA.
BNC + GABA – Up to 100 pounds, use ½ teaspoon dissolved in juice, in the morning and in the afternoon. If over 100 pounds, use 1 to 2 teaspoons of powder, in the morning and in the afternoon.

Brain Link – 2 to 3 scoops, in the morning and in the afternoon, depending on weight.

Glutamine Powder (1000 mg per scoop) – 1 scoop, twice daily, in water or juice OR

Glutamine capsules (500 mg) – 2 capsules, twice to three times daily.

Ginkgo – 1 (40 mg) capsule, twice daily.

Huperzine A* – 1 capsule, twice daily.

Pregnenolone – 10 to 50 mg daily, depending on your age, upon awakening in morning.

Deluxe Scavengers – 3 capsules, daily.

T-L Vite – 1 capsule, daily, with main meal. This formulation contains, in one capsule, all the vitamins needed for better brain function.

Mag Link – 1 to 2 tablets, twice to three times daily.

Phosphatidylserine – 1 (100 mg) capsule, one to three times daily, divided.

*Do not use Huperzine A if you have any heart or pulmonary problems, or if you are pregnant or lactating.

Carpal Tunnel Syndrome
Repetitive Stress Injury

Carpal tunnel syndrome (CTS) is a neuropathy caused by an entrapment and compression of the medial nerves as they pass through the carpal tunnel area of the wrist. This results in a loss of motor function, including pain, numbness, and tingling in the middle three fingers. Other clinical symptoms include a pins-and-needle sensation in the entire hand, sleep disturbances, and weakness progressing to atrophy centered around the hand and wrist. Warning signs include pain, numbness, a tingling or burning sensation, weakness or loss of grip strength, and loss of sleep due to discomfort.

Repetitive stress/strain injuries (RSI) have now become known as the workplace curse of the new millennium. RSI symptoms can include everything from neck and shoulder pain, to back strain, all caused by prolonged repetitive movements involved in certain occupations or recreational activities. Manual tasks that repeatedly flex and extend the wrist intensify CTS with swelling and by compressing the wrist nerves. RSI may hit abruptly or have a slow onset involving one or both hands. The nerves must receive proper nourishment, or the symptoms caused by the lack of nourishment cause the median nerve to short circuit, requiring you to seek treatment. Do not delay treatment; your thumb, index finger, and middle finger can atrophy the thenar (palm) muscle, rendering your hand *permanently useless.*

The standard medical treatments for CTS include cortisone injections and surgery to relieve the pressure on the nerve. Sometimes these treatments cause permanent disabilities, in addition to the consequences of failing to address a B6 deficiency. In one twelve-week study, twenty-two patients with CTS were given between 50 to 300 mg of B6. All but one of the thirty-nine affected hands responded to the B6 treatment—a 97.4 percent cure rate!

B6 works by correcting the function of the synovium, the sheath encompassing the tendons. B6 stimulates the body's production of cortisone, thus decreasing the swelling in the tendon sheath, which, in turn, releases the pressure on the median nerve. Hyaluronic acid, the lubricant inside joints and the carpal tunnel, needs B6 to be produced by the body.

Suggested Nutritional Support

Rodex B6 – 1 (150 mg), timed-release B6, daily.

DMSO or 5% MSM lotion – Apply topically to wrist, as needed, for swelling.

Mag Link – 2 tablets, twice daily, for muscle tension and strain.

Glucosamine – 500 mg capsule, three times daily.

PoweRelief* – 1 or 2 capsules, every 6 hours, as needed for pain.

Bromelain – 500 mg, twice daily, to support tissue repair and reduce swelling.

Ester C – 1,000 mg, morning and evening.

Magnetic wrist tube or wrap support – wear daily, as needed.

Mood Sync** – 1 capsule, twice daily, for mood support.

Ice Pack – At night, use an ice pack, such as SofTouch packs, to

---

*Do not use DLPA if you are taking MAO inhibitors or tricyclic antidepressants, have had a malignant melanoma, are pregnant or lactating, or if you have PKU.

**Do not take if you are taking an SSRI, tricyclic, or MAO inhibitor medications.

Symptoms of Chronic Emotional Fatigue and Chronic Stress Syndrome

1. Anxiety
2. Mood swings
3. Mental and physical fatigue
4. Sluggishness
5. Chronic muscle spasms
6. Uncertainty
7. Fear that comes and goes
8. Panic attacks
9. Sleep problems
10. Chronic digestive upset
11. Constant body aches and pains
12. Stiff neck and/or limited range of motion
13. Muscle jerks
14. Churning stomach
15. Eye strain
16. Loss of interest (in everything)
17. No sex drive
18. Pounding heart, skipped beats
19. Low self esteem
20. No confidence
21. Withdrawal
22. Sensitivity to bright lights
23. Sensitivity to noise, especially loud sounds
24. Depression
25. Tension headaches or other headaches
26. Constant stress
27. Blurred vision
28. Constant fear of failure
29. Feelings of helplessness and hopelessness
30. Feelings of guilt
31. As fatigued in the morning, upon awakening, as when you went to bed.
32. Apathy
33. Tension

reduce swelling and pain.

DHA – 2 capsules, daily, to enhance the production of antiin-flammatory eicosanoids, and reduce the production of pro-inflam-matory eicosanoids.

MSM – 750 mg, three times daily. MSM is a dry form of DMSO—dimethyl sulfoxide—a naturally occurring sulfur compound and nutrient. MSM reduces pain, improves blood supply, and lowers muscle spasms and inflammation involved in CTS.

Chronic Emotional Fatigue

Millions of people suffer from Chronic Emotional Fatigue (CEF) and Chronic Stress Syndrome (CSS). The complexities of these pervasive problems indicate the need for more extensive research, information, and patient education. CEF and Stress Syndrome are not psychiatric problems and cannot be addressed by treating with antidepressants, tranquilizers, or pain pills.

Because of the complex natures of chronic emotional fatigue and chronic stress syndrome, patients must understand how their brain and body store emotions. Emotions are simultaneously every-where in the body. Emotion-and stress-related thoughts always move in an upward direction, which increases or causes anxiety after an emotional experience.

Chronic emotional fatigue and stress syndrome do not hap-pen overnight. They accumulate over months or years from non-stop fatigue and stress exhaustion. The program outlined in this text helps you heal and gives you a key to unlock the door that leads you to health, happiness, and peace of mind. You must take one day at a time and be patient with yourself or with a loved one who is suffering.

Chronic emotional fatigue and chronic stress syndrome bring about an intense, painful, nagging loss of control that affects ev-ery nerve fiber in your brain and body. Few people recognize it or know that the many symptoms they dread are no more than the symptoms of constant, unrelenting chronic stress that leads to full-blown emotional fatigue. However, the knowledge and un-derstanding of what is happening to you is a very powerful healer.

Over the past twenty years, I have watched patients go from doctor to doctor, looking for a magic bullet they never find. A magic bullet does not exist. Chronic emotional fatigue can attack you as physical fatigue, or emotional fatigue. This constant feeling of anxiety, or mental fatigue, keeps you from being able to function on a daily basis. Emotional fatigue uses nervous energy and allows the chemicals produced by muscular fatigue, such as lactic acid, to collect throughout the body. This is one reason why anxious people often complain of aching legs, back, necks, and even arms. This kind of ache is so intense that standing for short periods of time causes very anxious or stressed people to look for some type of support to lean on, or to head straight home to bed. When pain and fatigue consume your body day and night, you lose the will to get better.

Stress causes chronic fatigue and chronic stress syndrome. Stress-induced illness is an accumulation of psychological and physical stress responses throughout your life. Emotional fatigue and chronic stress, in part, come from home or work. You are also influenced by your toxic environment, negative information, violence, crowded expressways, traumatic events, disease, or anything that makes you feel a loss of control over your life. Taking care of a loved one who is terminally ill, then experiencing the death, leaves you helpless, hopeless, and with feelings that consume your days and nights. Sometimes you even take on the same symptoms as the loved one you lost—even the same pain—but you have NO disease. What you feel is psychosomatic in nature: there is no pathology or disease. This does not mean there is no pain or fatigue. In fact, your body is overwhelmed with it. The longer you experience uncertainty, fear, stress, and anxiety, the more saturated your mind becomes. Mental stress then turns into physical symptoms.

Many patients in mid life tell me they begin to recall traumatic experiences from their childhood. This is not unusual when emotional fatigue controls your life. Each time you felt loss of control in your life experiences, it left an imprint on your brain. These experiences will resurface because they've been stored in your memory as negative, repressed emotions. Repressed emotions and stress are stored in every cell and every muscle of your body. This, alone, can cause symptoms of emotional fatigue, depression, and pain. Many sufferers live in their doctor's offices, having one test after another. They are ready and want to believe something is physically wrong with them. An actual illness would prevent their having to face the stress of dealing with and resolving their repressed negative experiences. When you live in the past, you are consumed by the past. When the past intrudes on the present, it brings forth a very powerful force of pain, emotional fatigue, and depression. For healing to occur, you must deal with all your feelings as they occur. Then you can let them go instead of recording them for later playback and more suffering.

Emotional fatigue and depression go hand in hand, because depression depletes the mind and body. Depression implies a downward direction, a depth out of which a depressed person must somehow drag him-or-herself. Most feel it as an endless struggle, but it does not have to be such. Do not struggle to lift yourself out of anything. Direct your energy to clearing yourself, not only from negative, depleting depression, but from chronic fatigue. Stop struggling and start healing.

Rushing around, trying to get yourself out of depression can increase your fatigue and depletion. Going out, meeting people, and keeping busy help. Too often, you feel better when you are out, but become depressed as soon as you see your home. You begin playing old tapes in your mind.

Please remember, recovery from depletion is gradual. You dipped deeply into your emotional reserves. It will take time for these reserves to be replenished, just as a wound takes time to heal. This means you must work with your feelings of depression. You must be prepared to take them with you, even though they press heavily on your heart, and you feel a load of lead in your lungs.

If your doctor suggests antidepressants, they are *not* the answer; they will *not* help. Tell your doctor you prefer using a natural alternative such as amino acids. Amino acids treat the problem, not just the symptoms. Orthomolecular therapists and doctors know how to treat chronic emotional fatigue. You must restore your immune system and balance your brain chemistry.

If you are willing to work on understanding that feelings of depression are a form of depletion, the temporary symptoms soon pass. Time and healing gradually recharge your batteries, especially after the age of forty. *Do not be impatient!*

Constant, anxious inward thinking in chronic emotional fatigue brings "brain drain"—mental fatigue. Thoughts slow down and thinking becomes an effort. In a chronically, emotionally drained person, thoughts come with a great deal of effort. It is almost as if each thought has to be worked through twice. These sufferers become easily confused, finding concentration and remembering arduous.

When mental fatigue and sensitization work together, they throw off frightening ideas that seem impossible. Do not let this disturb you, and don't use your energy fighting unwanted thoughts. Just let them flow so you can work to either resolve or let them go. If you fight them, you add more tension and make the thoughts seem even more important. What you make important is more difficult to forget. Do not fight to forget them, just tell yourself they are unimportant. See them for what they are—only thoughts. Work with them and, with time, they will dissolve.

Fatigue accentuates unreality. Fatigue of the eye muscles interferes with the functioning of the lens. Vision seems blurred, so you have difficulty focusing. You notice it more when looking from a near object to a distant one, or vice versa. Objects in bright sunlight seem as if they are in dark shadows. The sufferer complains that everything suddenly goes dark, provoking fear. But, these symptoms are only temporary. Because you do not understand that this black world is caused by eye-muscle fatigue, you panic. You add more stress and tension to your body, so it takes longer for the world to return to its normal brightness.

Can you see how important it is to understand the chronic fatigue progression? Most people do not know how fear and fatigue trick you into thinking the wrong things. Again, acceptance, staying in reality, letting your mind and body float, drift, and relax are the keys!

In many ways, suffering like yours is a marker. We learn by contrast. Until we know emotional pain, we never know the true meaning of peace, and God knows you have known pain. Later, when you are able to step back and look at your life, things take on a new meaning. The pain is not as intense, and you are able to understand physical and mental fatigue. Never regret what you have been through. Your journey was a learning experience. Starting now, this very moment—not tomorrow—try your best to accept it. Stop struggling and fighting the rain. When you stop the struggle, you gradually return to your old self but with more understanding and sensitivity. Your energy will come back, and you will, again, look forward to each day of life.

Chronic emotional fatigue attacks those who cannot express, sort out, or deal with stress, anxiety, depression, fear, or grief. Do not repress. *Express.* If someone is trying to take control of your life, declare yourself! *You* take control of your life. *Use health, happiness, and peace of mind as the keys to the best quality of life you've ever dreamed possible!*

Suggested Nutritional Support

DHEA – Upon arising, take 1 (25 mg) capsule, *if over 40;* 1 (50 mg) capsule, if over 60.

Brain Link Complex – 3 scoops, daily.

Or Use **T-L Vite** – 1 capsule with 2 Balanced Neurotransmitter Complex (BNC) capsules.

Deluxe Scavenger – 3 capsules, daily.

CoEnzyme Q10 – 50 mg, daily.

Mag Link – 2 tablets. If loose stools or diarrhea occurs, decrease by 1 tablet, or try spreading the interval(s) between doses.

Mood Sync* – 2 capsules, three times per day. If you feel more anxiety, add an Anxiety Control capsule in place of 1 Mood Sync.

Digestive enzyme (such as Super Digestaway and/or Pancreatin) – 1 with each meal.

Ester C – 2 (500 mg) capsules in the morning and in the evening.

Alpha KG – 1 capsule, three times daily.

Adenosine Monophosphate – 1 tablet, three times daily.

Mag Link – 2 tablets.

Chromium Picolinate – 1 (200 mcg) capsule.

5-HTP* – 1 (50 mg) capsule, 1 hour prior to bedtime.

Use the following supplements as needed.

Chronic pain – 2 PoweRelief** as needed, using up to 6 daily.

Irritable Bowel Syndrome – 1 Calm Colon, three times daily.

*Do not use if you are taking an SSRI drug.

**Do not use Tyrosine, Phenylalanine, or DLPA if you are pregnant or lactating, have PKU or if you use MAO inhibitors or tricyclic antidepressants, or if you have had a malignant melanoma.

Skin problems – Lysine 1,000 to 3,000 mg daily along with MSM cream or lotion.

Memory problems – Huperzine A***, 1 (50 mcg) capsule in the morning and in the evening.

Perimenopausal women – 2 Balanced Woman capsules, twice daily.

***Do not use if you have pulmonary or heart trouble or if you are pregnant or lactating, you should not use Huperzine.*

Chronic Pain

Chronic pain is America's most common, expensive, disabling, and overprescribed disorder. Research demonstrates that patients who suffer for long periods become very depressed. The longer you suffer, the greater the intensity of pain. Pain sends an estimated 120+ million Americans to doctors, pain clinics, and chiropractors, every year. Pain cripples our lives and drives millions to addictive prescription drugs and alcohol.

Every year, the American public spends 6 billion dollars for analgesics (painkillers) and therapies of every description, but they still experience pain. Pain is one of the most serious problems not only in the U.S., but in the world. Back pain afflicts 85 million, arthritis 56 million, migraines 30 million; and 900,000 live with the hell on earth of cancer pain.

There are no magic bullets, no miracle drugs, no overnight cures. If anyone tells you they have a cure for pain, run, don't walk away. If a physician tells you surgery is the answer, get a second opinion and then make sure they review all the potential postsurgical problems. If you are offered an array of medication, consider the long-term effects, because drugs treat only the symptoms. Your goal is to treat the source—your brain—the master controller that sends signals to every corner of the body!

Remember, whatever the brain tells the body to do, it does! Pain research at Johns Hopkins University indicates a great deal of chronic pain and depression reflects the patient's inability to produce enough of certain brain chemicals. This research points to new methods of treating pain and depression, without using harmful drugs.

Studies at other major universities have shown the brain does produce many hormone-like chemicals that have a close functional resemblance to morphine. These morphine-like chemicals are called endorphins (endogenous morphine) because they are produced by the body (endogenous), and are similar to morphine.

Endorphins regulate pain and control the transmission of pain signals. Endorphins are inhibitory neurotransmitters in the brain and nervous system. They slow down the transmission of pain information from the limbic system to the cortex. Endorphins and other neurotransmitters help link together the one-hundred-plus billion neurons of the human brain into an incredibly complex network. From this complex network comes our natural painkillers, endorphins. Endorphins have been shown to be more powerful than morphine. Are they the answer to pain control? Yes and no.

Endorphins are not drugs, but a simple nutritional amino acid, phenylalanine. The pain studies involved DL-Phenylalanine, or DLPA. DLPA is not a drug. It does not actually block pain, itself. DLPA works by protecting your own naturally produced endorphins, effectively extending their life spans in the nervous system. By extending their lifespans, pain relief results. DLPA is a natural healer. It helps the body heal itself. Depression loves pain, pain loves depression; but DLPA has the ability to elevate the brain chemistry so that you do not feel depressed and in more pain. DLPA can do this because it is an inhibitory neurotransmitter.

DLPA is now being used clinically throughout the U.S. in major pain clinics, for pain and depression. Millions of people suffering from pain do so because of stress. Stress energizes pain, pain fuels stress. We see patients every day taking a combination of pain medications and antidepressants for stress-induced pain. *Harrison's Principles of Internal Medicine* states 50 to 80% of all pain is stress induced. This means there is no pathology; the pain is there, but there is no disease.

Those who suffer from stress-induced pain are depressed and negative because they are low in 34 of the 36 neurotransmitters made from amino acids. Most amino acids, themselves, are pain-relievers, especially 5-HTP—a safe, natural way to boost serotonin levels. Serotonin is absolutely essential for smooth brain function. If you live with chronic pain, you are deficient in serotonin, and, therefore, are more sensitive to pain messages from the brain.

Suggested Nutritional Support

DLPA 750* – Take 5 minutes after meals, 3 times per day. Keep in mind DLPA takes from 2 days to 3 weeks to take effect. If your doctor has prescribed medication, you do not have to stop taking it. DLPA can greatly enhance the effectiveness of aspirins and analgesics.

Rodex B6 (time released) – 1 capsule, 150 mg, before breakfast.

Mag Link – 2 tablets mid-morning and 2 mid-afternoon. If no diarrhea or loose stools occur, try increasing to a total of six per day. Take to bowel tolerance, then decrease by 1.

Powerelief* – 2 caps, two to three times per day.

Boswella Plus – 1 or 2 capsule(s), mid-morning and mid-afternoon.

Mood Sync** – 2 capsules in the morning, and 2 in the evening.

Taurine 1000 – 1 capsule, three times per day.

TL Vite – 1 capsule with breakfast.

Or use **Brain Link** – 3 scoops in the morning.

GABA 375 or 750 – 1 capsule, two to three times per day.

Mobigesic – 1 tablet every 4 to 6 hours.

Bromelain – 2 capsules 500 mg in the morning, and 2 in the evening.

Ester C – 1000 mg, four times per day.

5-HTP** – Start with 1 (50 mg capsule or tablet) 30 minutes before bedtime; increase to 2, if needed.

OR use **Melatonin** – 1 (3 mg) capsule an hour before bed, for sleep.

Relaxation tape – Try to use a relaxation tape at least 30 minutes a day. If your muscles are relaxed, your muscles will not increase your pain with spasms.

---

*Do not use if you have PKU, have had a melanoma, are pregnant or lactating, or if you use MAO inhibitors or tricyclic antidepressants.
**Do not use if you are taking an SSRI, tricyclic, or MAO inhibitor antidepressant.

Depression

Depression is an intensely isolating experience that can lead to losing a positive self-image and self-worth. You feel lost and alone, and no matter how you try, you cannot seem to pull yourself up from the darkness. There is hope for the twenty million Americans suffering from chronic depression, the dark and lonely emotion.

Depression is very treatable without toxic antidepressant drugs. Antidepressants cause you to give up control and let the drugs block your feelings. Drugs cause you to live a passive existence. There is no such thing as a tranquilizer deficiency! The causes of depression include genetic, biological, personality, environmental, and nutrient deficiencies. Stress-related events may be the major cause of cell depression and events that occurred in early life can prime the limbic system for later depression.

Depression can coexist with other disorders both physical and psychological. Each disorder can feed off the other such as chronic pain, fibromyalgia, or headaches.

If you have a chemical imbalance causing your depression, you have a deficiency of norepinephrine or serotonin. These two neurotransmitters are the major neurotransmitters that control mood in the brain. Drugs work by manipulating these neurotransmitters usually by increasing the amounts of norepinephrine or serotonin.

Tyrosine, because of its role in assisting the body to cope physi-

Major Symptoms of Depression

- Passive negativity
- Oversleeping combined with chronic fatigue
- Constant indigestion
- Dry mouth
- Compulsive eating, especially carbohydrates
- Appetite loss or changes in eating patterns
- Constipation or diarrhea
- Inability to make decisions
- Loss of confidence or self esteem
- Frequent or unexplainable crying

ologically with stress and building the body's natural store of adrenaline, deserves to be called the stress amino acid. Stress exhaustion needs tyrosine which is converted to dopamine, norepinephrine, and epinephrine. The use of tyrosine in depression increases levels of serotonin and neurotransmitters. These help restore a sense of well-being.

Tyrosine was first used in psychiatry for medication-resistant depression. Dr. A. J. Gelenberg (1980), of the Department of Psychiatry at Harvard Medical School, used tyrosine to treat patients who presented with depression. These patients noted significant improvement with tyrosine.

5-HTP, or 5-Hydroxytryptophan boosts the serotonin levels in the brain and creates neurotransmitters that produce an inhibitory effect on the nervous system. 5-HTP is converted into serotonin in the brain. Serotonin soothes, calms, and gives you a warm feeling of contentment. If you have a deficiency of serotonin, symptoms of depression, obsessive-compulsive disorder, anxiety, pain, and migraines will be demonstrated. Both Mood Sync and Teen Link contain 5-HTP.

St. John's Wort (SJW) is known as the depression herb, and it has been used for centuries. SJW's effectiveness has been confirmed by multiple double-blind studies comparing SJW to tricyclic antidepressants such as Elavil and Tofranil. The effective dose is 300 mg, three times, a day. SJW inhibits the breakdown of neurotransmitters like serotonin and weakens inhibition of the enzyme MAO. SJW should not be used with phenylalanine or tyrosine.

People with allergies or high histamine levels will have chronic low-grade depression. Additionally for allergy sufferers, add 500 to 1,000 mg of methionine daily, divided doses, and BCAAs (Branched Chain Amino Acids), 500 to 1,000 mg, daily. These amino acids will help you feel better.

For information regarding SAMe, see methionine section.

Suggested Nutritional Support

Tyrosine 850* – For chronic depression, use 850 mg, twice daily.

B6 – 100 to 150 mg daily, preferably in timed-release form, such as

*Do not use if you have PKU, have had a melanoma, are pregnant or lactating, or if you use MAO inhibitors or tricyclic antidepressants.

Rodex B6.

GABA 750 – Use 1/2 capsule three times daily, divided and dissolved in water. GABA levels of those with depression are usually low. This information surfaced in a study done by F. Petty, M.D., of the Department of Psychiatry, Veterans Medical Center in Dallas.

Liquid Serotonin – 10 to 15 drops, 3 times daily, or as needed.

Mood Sync** – 1 or 2 capsules, twice to three times daily.

5-THP** – 2 at bedtime.

Methionine – 1,500 mg, three times daily with 2 BNC in the morning. *For information regarding SAMe, see methionine section.*

Children

For children *under 100 pounds*, use 500 mg tyrosine,* once daily with 50 mg B6. If *over 100 pounds*, use 500 mg tyrosine, twice daily with 50 mg B6.

HTP10** – 1 capsule, twice daily, if under 100 pounds. If over 100 pounds, use 2 HTP10, twice daily,

Or Use **Teen Link**** – 1 capsule, twice daily.

Teenagers

Teen Link** – 1 or 2 capsules, twice daily. Always start with 1 capsule twice daily, and see if that lifts the depression. Only if depression is not eased, increase to 2, twice to three times daily.

*Do not use if you have PKU, have had a melanoma, are pregnant or lactating, or if you use MAO inhibitors or tricyclic antidepressants.

**Do not use if you are taking an SSRI, tricyclic, or MAO inhibitor antidepressant.

Health Capsule Factoid

Sudden Withdrawal from Paroxetine (Paxil) may cause vertigo or dizziness, a new phenomenon of serotonin withdrawal syndrome. Acute sudden withdrawal from Paxil causes more withdrawal symptoms than other SSRI medications. Other withdrawal side effects include gastrointestinal problems that may persist as long as 21 days. The cause of these withdrawal symptoms is unknown.

Diabetes

Approximately 10 million Americans have diabetes. Diabetes is a chronic disorder of carbohydrate, fat, and protein metabolism. Diabetes occurs when the pancreas does not secrete enough insulin, or if the cells of the body become insulin resistant. As a result, blood sugar is unable to get into the cells. Diabetes can lead to multiple serious medical complications.

There are two basic types of diabetes: Type 1 and Type II. Patients with Diabetes Mellitus, or Type I, are insulin-dependent. This most often occurs in children and adolescents. Type II usually begins after the age of 40. Type II diabetics are non-insulin dependent, and comprise 90% of all diabetics.

According to Julian Whitaker, M.D. in his book *Reversing Diabetes*, some of his patients with Type I diabetes report having very stressful events in their lives that occurred six months to a year before they developed diabetes. Stress can alter the immune system, causing it to weaken. This predisposes an individual to the disease state, and often the onset of diabetes.

Suggested Nutritional Program

Always use capsule, powder, or liquid form for maximum absorption.

Anxiety Control 24 – 1 or 2 capsules, twice per day, or as needed to decrease stress and anxiety.

Chromium Picolinate – 600 mcg daily, divided to help regulate blood sugar and decrease insulin resistance.

Gymnema Sylvestre – 300 mg, three times daily, divided before meals. Gymnema Sylvestre is a herb that aids in controlling sugar uptake and cravings. It helps to maintain normal blood-glucose levels.

Mag Link – 2 tablets twice to three times daily. If loose stools occur, decrease the dose by 1, or try spreading out the interval between doses.

Vanadium – 100 to 150 mg per day, divided. Vanadium helps with blood glucose reduction. (You may have to cut back on your oral medications. Do this under the supervision of your physician.)

Carnitine – 2 (250 mg) capsules, twice per day. Carnitine is important in fat distribution in the body. It helps reduce cholesterol and triglyceride levels to normal in the body.

Fiber – helps keep blood sugar in the normal range. Use 2 tablespoons of Fortified Flax in any food or beverage. Fortified Flax provides 4600 mg of Omega 3 (good oil) needed on a daily basis.

Rodex B6 – 1 timed-release capsule in the morning.

Taurine – 500 mg capsule, twice daily, to aid the release of insulin.

Deluxe Scavenger (antioxidants) – 3 per day, divided. Deluxe Scavenger combines CoEnzyme Q10, beta-carotene, Vitamin C, Lemon bioflavonoids, rutin, Vitamin E, Selenium, Glutathione, NAC, riboflavin, P5'P, and Vitamin B6.

Vitamin C (Ester C) – 2,000 to 3,000 mg per day, divided. Vitamin C is vital for the repair of all body tissues and scavenger of free radicals in the body.

Vitamin E – 400 to 800 I.U. daily. Vitamin E is important for the circulation, heart, neurological functions, and scavenging free radicals.

Manganese – 15 mg daily. Manganese is important for pancreas repair.

CoEnzyme Q10 – 80 to 120 mg (in capsules) per day. CoQ10 supports the immune system, helps provide increased oxygen to the heart and body, and acts as a protective factor for the heart.

Alpha-Lipoic Acid (ALA) – 300 mg, twice daily; ALA is especially important for diabetic neuropathy.

Gymnema Sylvestre (GS) – 600 mg, three times daily. GS is a sugar blocker and helps regenerate the beta cells of the pancreas.

Eat as many fruits and vegetables as possible. This increases fiber which helps stabilize blood sugar, and reduces the need for insulin.

Amino Acids and the Elderly

Many factors contribute to how quickly we age. The combined effects of genetic inheritance, health habits, medical history, life-style, sociocultural background, and environment all play a part in our aging. Many of the elderly do not take the time to

Ingestion (%) of R.D.V. in People Over 60

	M	F		M	F
Vitamin B6	66	72	Vitamin D	51	62.5
Vitamin B12	19	31	Calcium	20	35
Folic Acid	54	72	Zinc	40	67

cook nutritional foods. Therefore, they deplete their immune system and illness prevails.

Senior citizens are more prone to fatigue, dizziness, and falls, as their muscles do not respond as quickly as they did when they were younger. Sudden movements or exertion can increase the probability of falls.

The heart muscle begins to wear out from the stress of everyday life. The muscle becomes less elastic with age from exposure to free radicals found in air, sun, and environment. Cardiac output

Function, Cognition, and Behavior Influenced by Nutrients

Nutrient	*Influence*
Taurine	Seizures
Carnitine	Cognition, depression
Phenylalanine	Catecholamines, dopamine, depression
5-HTP (Tryptophan)	Sleep, serotonin, neurotransmitters
Thiamin (B1)	Carbohydrate sensitivity
Riboflavin (B2)	Neurotransmitter control, neuropathy
Niacin (B3)	Dementia
Pyridoxine (B6)	Neurotransmitter cofactor
Cobalamin (B12)	Dementia
Folic Acid	Dementia
Choline	Memory, Acetylcholine synthesis
Inositol	Peripheral neuropathy
Pantothenic Acid	Fatigue
Vitamin E	Parkinson's Disease
Iron	Neurophysiological problems
Magnesium	Sleep disturbances, nervous exhaustion
Zinc	Smell, taste
Copper	Neurotransmitter control, RBC formation

is reduced due to thickening and hardening of the heart valves and chambers. The overall consequences reduce oxygen delivery to the cells. In addition, plaques of fat build up in our blood vessels and arteries.

Elasticity loss in the lungs reduce vital capacity. Damage from free radicals stiffens the exchange sacs called alveoli. As a result, the air exchange is compromised, affecting the health of the body tissues.

As a person ages, their ability to digest proteins diminishes. The amount of stomach acid-and protein-digesting enzymes decreases. Up to 30% of people over 60 do not secrete any stomach acid. Since most people over 60 have a decreased ability to digest proteins, and proteins are broken down into amino acids, then supplementation with amino acids will provide a base to cover the essential amino acids needed by the body.

The digestion and elimination process slows down as we age. Poor appetite is a common complaint, due to many factors. Salivary secretion decreases by 50 to 60%. Loss of teeth, or gum disease, makes chewing more difficult and painful. Constipation may result from decreased fluid intake, lack of fiber, little or no exercise, and decreased intestinal motility.

Probably one of the most apparent changes occurs in the skin. The skin loss or resiliency and wrinkling becomes very evident. The skin becomes drier, thinner, more fragile, and less elastic.

The bones begin to break down through bone demineralization, reduced exercise and activity, and loss of calcium from kidneys and intestines. The loss of height becomes apparent in many seniors. The mineral loss in bones makes the bones more fragile and brittle. Sometimes the bones break, causing a fall.

Nutritional status influences all parts of the nervous system. The neurotransmitters regulate the physiological processes, and the way the brain processes information relates to our nutritional status. In several studies done on individuals 65 and over, the results indicate cognitive tasks corresponded to the nutritional status of the individual.

Alterations in psychological and neurophysiological performances occur when a person is deprived of, or low in, the B vitamins. As an example, acetylcholine derives from the B complex vitamin, choline. Inadequate amounts of choline can affect the synthesis, release, and metabolism of acetylcholine, and alter nerve function. Serotonin, an inhibitory neurotransmitter derived from tryptophan, decreases with age. Conversely, the catecholamine family—epinephrine, norepinephrine, and the neurotransmitters derived from phenylalanine or tyrosine—decreases with aging. These changes can produce mood swings, depression, and sleep-pattern alterations. The nutritional status based on a person's unique genetic needs, determines cognitive and behavioral functioning.

In the past decade researchers have realized the relationship between the activity and function of the nervous system to the availability and metabolic activity of various nutrient-derived substances, including amino acids, vitamins, minerals, essential fatty acids, and other conditionally essential nutrients such as carnitine, taurine, and glutamine.

Suggested Nutritional Support *(Over age 60)*

For all seniors, *always use powder, liquid or capsule form. Never take in tablet form,* as tablets do not break down as readily, so absorption is impaired.

BNC Plus – 1 teaspoon, twice daily, in fruit juice. ⎫ Use all three

B Complex – 1 capsule, twice per day. ⎬ together **OR** use Brain

TL Vite – 1 capsule in the morning, ⎭ Link

Or Use **Brain Link Complex** – 1 scoop in the morning, and 1 in afternoon.

Deluxe Scavenger (antioxidants) – 1 capsule, three times per day.

CoEnzyme Q10 – 50 mg capsule, once per day.

Mag Link – 2 in the morning, and 2 in the evening.

Cal, Mag, Zinc – 4 capsules at bedtime.

5-HTP* – For sleep, 1 or 2 capsules an hour before bedtime, with a piece of fruit. Always start with 1 capsule, increase to 2, if needed.

Or Use **Melatonin** – For sleep, 1 (3 mg) capsule, an hour before bed.

Liquid Serotonin – 10 to 20 drops, as needed, for agitation or insomnia.

DHEA – 1 (50 mg) capsule upon arising in the morning.

Pregnenolone – 1 (50 mg) capsule, upon arising in the morning.

*Do not use if you are taking an SSRI, tricyclic, or MAO inhibitor antidepressant.

Fortified Flax – For constipation, start with 1 teaspoon twice per day, dissolved in fruit juice. Increase up to 1 tablespoon, if needed; *Or Use* **Magnesium Chloride Liquid** – Use ½ to 1 teaspoon dissolved in fruit juice, once or twice per day, as needed for constipation.

Phosphatidylserine – 100 mg, three times per day, if cognitive functions are deteriorating.

Huperzine – 50 mcg capsule, twice daily to increase memory and concentration. *Do not use Huperzine if any heart or pulmonary problems exist, or if you are pregnant or lactating.*

Grief

The symptoms of grief are many, and the grieving process is a slow and painful process. The symptoms of grief behavior are extensive. These behaviors can be described under four general categories.

A) Feelings
B) Physical symptoms
C) Cognitive
D) Behaviors

A person in grief experiences a wide range of mental symptoms and feelings including depression, denial, anger, anxiety, fear, uncertainty, etc.

Grieving Process

For those who cared for a sick relative, grief and depression hit harder and longer. A study sponsored by the National Institute of Mental Health found 30% of caregivers suffer from clinical depression or anxiety while their loved one is alive. Four years later, 25% still suffered symptoms. Of those 25% still suffering, 50% experienced sleeplessness, 61% depression, 41% back pain, and 24% stomach problems. Only 10% of non-caregiving *relatives were depressed for four years after death.*

Physical Sensations Most Commonly Experienced from Grief

- Hollowness in the stomach
- Tightness in the chest
- Tightness in the throat
- Oversensitivity to noise, bright lights, and certain smells (such as hospitals)
- Unreality
- Breathlessness or shortness of breath
- Muscle weakness
- Fatigue
- Dry mouth
- Waking up several times nightly
- Appetite changes
- Chronic pain
- Headaches

Appetite disturbance presents a major problem and can cause long-term illness, if not addressed properly and corrected. In grief, your neurotransmitter level will be very low from the prolonged stress and anxiety. Grief can cause fuzzy or irrational thinking, as well as avoidance behaviors. Many people refuse to let go or "close the casket," and go on with their life. Staying in the past with a loved one can cause anxiety and phobias as well as physical illnesses.

Note: Find a therapist you can talk to and with whom you feel comfortable sharing your feelings. See him/her at least weekly through your acute stage, then on a monthly basis for the first year, and then as needed. Do not repress your feelings. Allow them to flow. If you took care of a loved one during a long illness, you can take on their symptoms which can include fear, depression, as well as their physical pain. Close the casket. Say good-bye, and let them go. Otherwise, your healing cannot begin.

Suggested Nutritional Support
Adults

Mood Sync* – 1 or 2 capsules, twice to three times per day, in acute stage; and then 1 to 2, twice per day, as maintenance. *Do not use if you are taking an SSRI antidepressant.*

OR Use **Tyrosine**** – 500 mg, 2 to 3 times daily, spread throughout the day.

B6 – 50 mg in the morning.

Brain Link Complex – 1 serving in the morning.

OR Use **TL-Vite** – 1 in the morning with breakfast.

5-HTP* – 1 (50 mg) capsule, 1 hour prior to bedtime. Do not use if you are taking an SSRI antidepressant.

Liquid Serotonin – Use 10 to 15 drops as needed throughout the day.

Mag Link – 2 tablets, twice daily.

Anxiety Control – For acute episodes of anxiety, 1 or 2 capsules twice to three times daily, divided, as needed.

Taurine 1000 – 1 capsule, twice daily.

Children

Brain Link Complex – use 1/2 scoop in juice, in the morning.

Tyrosine* – 200 to 500 mg depending on weight, daily. Under 50 pounds, use 200 mg.

Liquid Serotonin – Use 6 to 10 drops, as needed, throughout the day.

Anxiety Control 24 – 1 capsule, mid-morning, afternoon, and 30 minutes before bedtime.

Taurine 1000 – 1 capsule daily.

Teenagers

Teen Link** – Use 1 or 2 capsules, twice daily.

Brain Link Complex – 1 serving in the morning, and 1 in the evening.

Taurine 1000 – 1 capsule, twice daily.

- Avoid sugar and do not use alcohol for depression.
- Avoid prolonged periods in dark rooms or rooms with drapes closed except when sleeping.

*Do not use if you have PKU, have had a melanoma, are pregnant or lactating, or if you use MAO inhibitors or tricyclic antidepressants.

**Do not use if you are taking an SSRI, tricyclic, or MAO inhibitor antidepressant.

Grief from Pet Loss

Your pets become part of your family, and when their lives come to an end, you can experience deep feelings of grief and loss. There is no set time for your grief, or for how long it will last. Don't be ashamed to express your feelings of loss. Your pet intertwined with the daily rhythms of your life, especially when you first came home, at meals, and at bedtime. You experience the same deep, lost, and lonely feelings you do with a human loss. When a beloved pet dies, part of your lifestyle is lost. All that your pet symbolized is lost—comfort, love, companionship, security, and joy.

Pets accept you unconditionally. They allow you to express any emotion. They don't judge, or criticize; they just love and accept. When the loss occurs, many of us feel confused by the deep level of grief, because your pet was part of your family and lived each hour of each day to give you love. Don't suppress your feelings. Allow them to flow so you can put closure on your loss, and allow the healing process to begin. Use the nutritional support program outlined, as long as needed. For special help, contact the Delta Society at 1-800-869-6898; they are available 24 hours, every day. They specialize in counseling those who have lost a pet and need assistance with their grief.

Headaches

Headache is the number-one complaint of the American public. Consumers spend approximately 6 billion dollars per year on pain medications and over-the-counter formulas for relief. It is estimated that yearly approximately 90% of men and 95% of women suffer from headaches painful enough to send them to doctors' offices. The source of the headaches is not located in the brain, itself, as there are no sensory nerves in the brain. Pain produced inside the skull is rare and usually due to tumors or other disorders; the pain is a secondary symptom. Most headache pain originates *outside* the skull in the nerves leading to the muscles and blood vessels around the face, scalp, and neck.

The most common types of headaches include migraine, tension or muscle contraction, and cluster. Often, a person can experience a combination of headaches. But headaches may also be caused by other underlying problems, such as sinus or allergy.

Food or stress can trigger migraines. Migraines are often called the avoidance headache. Migraine headaches produce a throbbing pain on one side of the head, but the pain can spread to the entire head. Often nausea and sometimes vomiting occur. Visual symptoms are common. Facial tingling or numbness may occur. Other symptoms include extreme sensitivity to noise and lights. Usually the attacks last from 4 to 72 hours without treatment, and commonly interfere with normal activity to some extent. Migraine sufferers may look pale and feel cold. Sometimes the victim gets a forewarning of an attack with malaise, fatigue, and mood changes. It is not uncommon for the sufferer to feel exhausted and mentally foggy for hours after an attack.

Headache triggers include:
- Stress, anxiety, anger, or depression.
- Menstruation, oral contraceptives, or hormone-replacement drugs.
- Foods such as dairy, MSG, eggs, anything pickled, alcohol (beer or red wine), coffee, teas, chocolate, wheat, cheese, or tomatoes are the most common. But any food can be a culprit. Explore food allergies as a contributing cause. There are lab tests for differentiating foods, or you can do a food-elimination diet.
- Environmental substances such as perfumes, paint, new carpet, glues, fumes, etc.
- Missed or delayed meals.
- Flickering fluorescent lights, sunlight.
- Time-zone changes.
- Holidays and travel.
- Strong smells.
- Loud noises.
- Bone structure misalignment and muscle spasms with trigger points.
- Alteration of sleep-wake cycle, such as sleep deprivation or excesses.

- Certain drugs.

Tension or muscle-contraction headaches are probably the most common form of headaches. Tension headaches account for 75% of all headaches, and are usually a response to stress, fatigue, or environmental factors; they can even start after a stressful event. The pain in the head results from muscle contractions of the head, neck, back, or facial muscles. Pain is often felt in the forehead, extending up from the base of the skull. The muscles of the upper back or neck contract, causing the pain to *refer* to the head. This is frequently described as a tight feeling, like a band or vise around the head. The neck and shoulders often feel sore, and the person can develop trigger points in the muscles. Trigger points are sore, tender points that form scar tissue within the muscle. The trigger point causes the muscle to go into contraction from stress, anxiety, overuse, poor posture, or staying in same position for an extended period of time. The headaches can become chronic and occur daily. Headaches can last only a few minutes, but usually last several days. Nausea is uncommon with muscle-contraction headaches, and usually do not limit activities as do migraines. But muscle-contraction headaches can make you feel that you are going crazy from the pain. The chronic muscle-contraction headache can bring on depression, anxiety, and sleep problems. Massage with deep-tissue work sometimes benefits. But if the muscle does not let go, it may be necessary to have trigger point injections to break up a headache.

Cluster headaches cause very severe one-sided head pain. Usually the pain centers in the eye. Other symptoms include excessive tearing, drooping eyelid, stuffy or runny nose, all on the side of the pain. Restlessness is a common symptom. The pain can be so severe that the sufferer paces or bangs their head against the wall to contend with the headache. Cluster headache attacks usually last 30 to 90 minutes, but they can last hours. The sufferer generally has recurrent attacks over a month to three months, with the headaches occurring during an active phase once or twice daily, or every other day. Then the headaches do not recur for several months to years. There is no known cause for cluster headaches.

About 90% of headaches are due to the aforementioned. Other most common causes of headaches include the following.

- Sinus headache. Due to increased pressure in the sinus cavities; often a sinus infection. Sinus headaches last until the sinuses drain. A sinus infection should be treated with antibiotics.

- Temporomandibular Joint Dysfunction (TMJ). Usually occurs in the *temple,* ear, or cheek regions of the head. Caused by clenching of the jaws, or grinding of the teeth. (Usually at night or from abnormalities of the jaw joint itself. Stress intensifies TMJ pain).
- Glaucoma. Increased intraocular (eye) pressure. Acute glaucoma may cause a throbbing pain around or behind the eye, or in the forehead. Eye redness and vision of halos or rings around lights may occur with glaucoma.
- Hypertension. Increased blood pressure; can contribute to a headache.
- Strokes, aneurysms and brain hemorrhages. A severe headache of sudden onset associated with stupor, or other neurological symptoms, demands prompt medical evaluation.
- Head trauma can cause pain, and can reflect serious damage ranging from fractured skull to internal bleeding.
- Occipital neuralgia headache. Occurs mainly in senior citizens. Symptoms include jabbing pain in the back of the head and neck, tenderness in neck and shoulder area.
- Other miscellaneous causes of headache include eyestrain, allergies, dental problems, dehydration, systemic infections, caffeine withdrawal, meningitis, brain swelling, and intense physical exertion.

If you have persistent pain that does not respond to rest and treatment, consult a physician. *If you experience a headache accompanied by severe pain, drowsiness, confusion, mood swings, visual disturbances, weakness or paralysis, consult a physician immediately.*

Suggested Nutritional Support for Headaches

Powerelief* – 1 or 2 caps every 4 to 6 hours, as needed, for relief. Powerelief combines DLPA, Boswella, GABA, Passion Flower, Magnesium, and B6.

DLPA 750* – 1 or 2 capsules, twice per day.

Mobigesic – 1 tablet, three times per day.

Boswella (300 mg) – 1 or 2, twice per day. Boswella is a herb

---

*Do not use if you have PKU, have had a melanoma, are pregnant or lactating, or if you use MAO inhibitors or tricyclic antidepressants.

from India, used for inflammation or swelling.

Anxiety Control 24 – 2 capsules, twice to three times per day.

Mag Link – 4 to 6 tablets per day, divided. If loose stools occur, then decrease by 1.

Mood Sync** – 1 or 2 capsules, two to three times daily, if you are depressed with a headache.

Feverfew – 1 capsule, twice per day, for prevention of migraines or to extend the life of DLPA.

Alka-Seltzer Gold – 2 tablets dissolved in a glass of water at onset of a migraine headache. Often, this brings immediate relief for migraine headaches triggered by allergic reactions to food or chemical substances. The Alka-Seltzer Gold helps to neutralize the allergic mechanism, and prevents the migraine from becoming full blown.

Riboflavin – 400 mg, daily, for prevention or reduction of migraines.

Accuband Magnets – Use on trigger points on the neck and upper back to relieve pain. Accubands are tiny, powerful magnets about the size of the top of a pencil eraser. They are applied with a small adhesive patch. These tiny magnets begin to ease pain immediately.

B Complex – 1 capsule in the morning.

Mobisyl Creme – Apply to neck and back once or twice per day.

NAC – For sinus congestion/headache, 1 (600 mg) capsule, twice daily.

- Elevate head above waist.
- Apply icepack to base of neck and on upper shoulders for 20 minutes at a time, then off for 30 minutes. Repeat as needed. (Try the SofTouch icebag—comes in its own cover, ready to use, and reusable. SofTouch packs are both freezeable and microwavable).
- Avoid heating pad for muscle-contraction or migraine headaches.
- For sinus headache, apply hot, moist towels or apply specially designed moist heating pad to the sinuses to facilitate sinus drainage.

**Do not use if you are taking an SSRI, tricyclic, or MAO inhibitor antidepressant.

- Massage to neck and shoulders can help relieve headache.
- Consider medical evaluation and trigger point injections, if headache persists.

Heart Disease

Heart disease or coronary heart disease (CHD) is the number one killer of Americans, and causes half the deaths in the U.S. today. An estimated 57 million Americans are afflicted with some type of heart disease. Heart disease claims over 720,000 people each year.

Risk factors include the following.

- Male gender, or postmenopausal women
- Genetics, history of heart disease in family
- Age
- High blood cholesterol
- Hypertension or high blood pressure
- Smoking
- Excess weight
- Lack of exercise
- Stress

Your sex, family history, and age pose risk factors beyond your control. But the other risk factors you *can* control. The most dangerous are high cholesterol, hypertension, and smoking. Each risk factor increases the risk of having a heart attack 2 to 3 fold, and all the risk factors compound each other dramatically.

Studies have shown that high cholesterol levels are directly proportional to your risk of heart attack. Diet is the next highest component that determines your cholesterol level. Dean Ornish, M.D., has proven cholesterol and your risk of heart disease can be dramatically changed with dietary and lifestyle changes, and love. Be aware, if you do not eat enough fat or cholesterol, the body increases the production of cholesterol in the liver. The body interprets the reduction of fats or cholesterol in the diet to a time of famine or starvation. This causes insulin to activate HMG Co-A reductase, an enzyme in the liver, to manufacture more cholesterol than is required by the body from sugars and carbohydrates.

Cholesterol lowering drugs work by inhibiting the HMG Co-A. Many cholesterol-lowering medications also lower the CoEnzyme Q10 level and can cause liver damage. This can put you at higher risk for having a heart attack. CoQ10 is an enzyme necessary for cell oxygenation, and is essential for health of all tissues and organs in the body. As we age, the CoQ10 level drops dramatically. CoQ10 helps protect against heart attacks, relieves angina, boosts the immune system, lowers blood pressure, is an antioxidant, and helps periodontal disease.

Hypertension or high blood pressure afflicts 35 million, or 1 in 6 Americans. If hypertension is present, the likelihood of CAD is 3 to 5 times higher than if the person has normal blood pressure. It is important that you have your blood pressure checked by a health care professional, at least twice yearly.

Smoking is the third controllable risk factor. Quit! A complete nutritional program is outlined in our *Breaking Your Prescribed Addiction* book. Your risk of a heart attack one year after you quit smoking is just 10% greater than the nonsmoker; after 5 years of abstinence, your risk factor becomes the same.

Suggested Nutritional Support

Carnitine – 1,000 to 3,000 mg per day, divided, for high cholesterol and triglycerides. Carnitine also increases the HDL (good) cholesterol. Immediately after a heart attack, supplement with 2 grams of carnitine to facilitate expansion of the heart muscle again. Continue carnitine at the 2 gram level. This helps reduce heart muscle damage while reducing angina and arrhythmias (abnormal heart rhythms).

Taurine – 1,000 mg, three times daily. Taurine is the most abundant amino acid in heart tissues. Taurine increases left ventricle function without changing the blood pressure, and helps balance the calcium and potassium in the heart.

Mag Link – 4 to 6 tablets per day, divided. If loose stools occur, decrease the dose by 1, or try spreading out the interval between doses. If you have CAD or hypertension, you are deficient in magnesium. Magnesium is nature's muscle relaxant, and is vital to a healthy heart. Mag Link is a magnesium chloride, the same form of magnesium found in the body; absorption and tolerance are best with this form of magnesium.

Chromium Picolinate – 200 mcg, per day. Chromium helps lower total cholesterol and triglycerides, while raising HDL cholesterol.

Vitamin E – 400 to 800 I.U., per day. Vitamin E is an antioxidant. Recent studies demonstrated a lower risk of fatal heart attack, if Vitamin E is taken daily.

DHEA – 25 to 50 mg per day, upon arising in the morning, on an empty stomach. (Have your physician check your DHEA sulfate level to obtain a starting point, and then have it checked 2 to 3 months after starting DHEA). In patients with CAD, the blood levels of DHEA have been very low; i.e., DHEA sulfate level of 4 (normal is 250—900).

CoEnzyme Q10 – 100 mg, per day, for CHD or hypertension. For congestive heart disease, increase CoEnzyme Q10 to 300 to 500 mg, per day, plus magnesium and B6.

Deluxe Scavenger – 3 per day divided. Deluxe Scavengers are a combination formula comprising CoEnzyme Q10, beta-carotene, Vitamin C, Lemon bioflavonoids, rutin, Vitamin E, Selenium, Glutathione, NAC, riboflavin, P5'P, and Vitamin B6.

Ester C – 2,000 to 5,000 mg per day, divided.

Garlic – 1,500 to 3,000 mg, divided. Garlic is an alternative to aspirin therapy. Ajoene, a component of garlic, is at least as potent as aspirin.

Folic acid – 400 to 800 I.U., daily. Folic acid is necessary for the proper metabolism of homocysteine. Excess homocysteine causes arterial plaque buildup.

Anxiety Control 24 – 1 or 2 capsules, twice or three times daily, as needed for anxiety or stress.

Rodex B6 – 150 mg capsule in the morning, for hypertension and congestive heart failure.

Hawthorn – 1 to 1.5 grams freeze-dried berries, three times daily. Hawthorn improves the circulation of blood to the heart by dilating blood vessels and relieving arterial spasms.

DHA – 2 capsules, twice daily. DHA, omega-3 fatty acids, decreases blood-platelet stickiness, lowers triglycerides, and lowers blood pressure.

Arginine – 1000 mg, twice daily. Arginine assists arterial blood vessels to release nitric oxide and it improves the blood vessels' abilities to dilate. Take Arginine with 1000 mg of lysine, twice daily, if you have problems with herpes outbreaks.

Herpes

Herpes has become a major social disease. Herpes attacks are characterized by clusters of clear, fluid-filled vesicles on the genitalia or face, accompanied by severe pain and itching. Once a person becomes infected with the herpes virus, rarely will the virus become extinct. The virus rests dormant in the body after the initial infection. When it reactivates as a result of stress, such as emotional upset, sunburn, etc., the virus produces an outbreak. Stress causes reemergence of the virus, and changes the balance of the amino acids arginine and lysine.

Keeping the balance of lysine to arginine at the right levels prevents replication of the herpes virus, and keeps it in check. Lysine is relatively easy to get in the diet, and most people consume ten times the minimum. However, vegetarians tend to have low lysine levels. A key to keeping herpes under control is to watch the ratio lysine-to-arginine foods. You must find the proper balance for you by trial and error. Avoid arginine-rich foods: chocolate, carob, coconut, oats, peanuts, soybeans, wheat germ, gelatin. Increase lysine foods: beef, chicken, lamb, milk, cheese, beans and brewer's yeast. In addition, take lysine supplementation in amounts of 500 to 1,500 mg per day.

Suggested Nutritional Support

Lysine – 500 to 1,500 mg per day as maintenance. During acute outbreaks, increase the lysine up to 3,000 mg, per day, and add another 1,000 mg of Vitamin C (Ester C).

Ester C with Bioflavonoids – 500 mg, three times per day.

Anxiety Control 24 – 1 or 2 capsules, twice per day. During an acute outbreak, increase to three times per day.

B Complex – 1 capsule, daily.

Lysine Cream – Apply to sores at onset, and repeat three to four times per day.

Powerelief* – 1 or 2 capsules, twice per day, as needed for pain. Powerelief contains DLPA, boswella, GABA, magnesium, and B6.

Vitamin E – 400 I.U. capsule, daily.

Zinc – 30 mg per day for acute outbreak until healed; then 15 mg per day for maintenance. Zinc is important to skin.

Ice Cube – If you feel tingling on an area around your mouth, apply an ice cube to the area for 5 minutes, then off for 5 to 10 minutes; repeat several times daily. This interrupts the viruses replication cycle, and may prevent a blister formation.

*Do not use if you are pregnant or lactating, have PKU or if you use MAO inhibitors or tricyclic antidepressants, or if you have had a malignant melanoma.

Irritable Bowel Syndrome (IBS)

An estimated 20% of the American population suffers from Irritable Bowel Syndrome (IBS), a common functional bowel disorder for which there is no reliable medical treatment. IBS is a disturbance of the intestines, resulting in diarrhea, abdominal pain, and/or constipation. Patients suffering from IBS have increased sensitivity, not only to painful distentions in the small bowel and colon, but to normal intestinal functions as well. Stress, anxiety, or any type of emotional conflict will provoke symptoms of IBS. IBS responds to psychological, physiological, or dietary influences on the brain and body.

In his book, *The Second Brain*, Michael Gershon, M.D., Columbia-Presbyterian Medical Center in Bronx, New York, established that the stomach has a brain that functions independently. This second brain is located in the gut, and contains neurons, neurotransmitters, and proteins. According to Dr. Gershon, this may be why patients suffer from ulcers, chronic abdominal pain, gastrointestinal disorders such as colitis, and from nervous-stomach butterflies caused by anxiety or panic.

The gut's brain, known as the enteric nervous system, resides in the tissues that line the digestive organs. Dr. Gershon reports the gut contains 100 million neurons, as well as nearly every major substance found in the brain. This enteric nervous system also comprises major neurotransmitters such as GABA, neuropeptides, and enkephalins. As a second brain, it operates independently of the central nervous system; however, it interacts very closely with the body's other brain because of its connection with the vagus nerve. The vagus nerve can receive anxiety-, fear-, and panic-related stimulation from the limbic system in the head brain. Repressed anger, hostility, or traumatic episodes can cause intestinal malfunction in the form of diarrhea. When the mind suffers, the body cries, and the entire nervous system responds with all the symptoms of IBS. People with multiple food sensitivities often experience symptoms of IBS. The primary offenders include dairy, wheat, and eggs. Other irritants involve coffee, corn, tea, citrus, some grains, and raw fruit. Once a person knows their food sensitivities, they can find useful fiber sources. Given the large number of people with wheat sensitivity, they can find relief with daily doses of the pleasant-tasting fortified flax. Fortified flax is rich in omega-3s, magnesium, fiber, and potassium.

Suggested Nutritional Support

Calm Colon – 1 capsule, three times daily. Calm Colon, a Chinese herbal formula, is the only clinically proven herbal support formula for IBS, and is described in *JAMA*.

Mag Link – 1 tablet, three times daily.

Anxiety Control – 2 capsules, as needed for stress and anxiety. If you have a problem with depression and anger, use Mood Sync; 1 capsule, four times daily.

Fortified Flax – 1 heaping teaspoon in the morning and in the evening.

Digestive Enzymes such as Super Digestaway – 1 with each meal.

Ginger – Use 1 or 2 capsules for upset stomach, as needed.

Alka-Seltzer Gold – Use 2 tablets, dissolved in water, as needed for food reactions, bloating, or upset stomach.

Mint Tea (such as peppermint) – after meals, to aid digestion.

GABA 375 – Mix 1 capsule with a small amount of water and drink if your stomach is upset from stress or anxiety. The GABA helps calm the receptors in your stomach.

Insomnia

Sleep disorders affect about 80 million people in the U.S. NIH reports 18 to 20% of the American public suffers from insomnia. Insomnia is the perception or complaint of poor-quality, or inadequate, sleep. There are several forms of insomnia—the ability to fall asleep when you first go to bed; or constantly waking up during the night and being unable to go back to sleep. Waking up in the early morning, unable to return to sleep, in most cases is due to anxiety. Insomnia can be the result of varied causes, including pain, anxiety, depression, grief, stress, fear, caffeine consumption, stimulant drug use, and certain psychoactive drugs.

Causes of Ongoing Insomnia

- Advanced age (>60 years)
- Female gender
- History of depression
- Stress/anxiety
- Medical problems
- Use of certain medications
- Chronic pain

Insomniacs spent over 600 million dollars for prescription sleep products in 1999, and this grows at a rate of 20% per year. The National Sleep Foundation found, through a Gallup Survey, that approximately 50% of all Americans have trouble sleeping. At some point during our lives, up to 50% of Americans have at least one bout of chronic insomnia, but only 20% go to a doctor for treatment.

Many women with PMS, or those approaching menopause, can experience interrupted sleep patterns due to hormonal imbalances. Millions of people suffer from a condition known as restless leg syndrome, or leg cramps. This condition, caused by a deficiency of magnesium, does not allow the muscles to relax, so they twitch and jerk all night. *Magnesium deficiency can cause insomnia.* Sleep apnea is a major problem and should be addressed by a physician who specializes in sleep disorders. If you have a problem with insomnia, do not consume any caffeinated coffee or beverage after 2 P.M.

Causes of Short-Term and Intermittent Insomnia

- Stress
- Environmental noise
- Temperature extremes
- Change in sleep environment
- Sleep/wake schedule problems
- Shift work
- Jet lag
- Medication side effects

Suggested Nutritional Support

5-HTP* – 1 (50 mg) capsule, 30 minutes prior to bed, to elevate your serotonin level. Increase to 2, if needed.

Mag Link – 2 tablets, twice to three times daily. Take to bowel tolerance, then decrease by one.

Melatonin – Start with a 2 mg capsule, 30 minutes prior to bedtime. Use melatonin *only* if you are over 30. If you experience weird dreams or nightmares, you are taking too large a dose.

Anxiety Control – 2 capsules, approximately 30 minutes prior to bedtime. If you wake up after a few hours, take an additional AC.

Mood Sync* – 1 or 2 capsules, two to three times daily.

Sedaplus – 1 or capsules, approximately 30 minutes prior to bedtime. Sedaplus is an herbal compound effective for sleep.

Powerelief** – 2 capsules, 30 minutes prior to bed, if you suffer from pain.

Mobigesic – 1, as needed for pain during the night.

MSM cream (10%) or lotion (5%), *or* **Mobisyl** – Rub on painful areas to reduce pain.

Other Therapies

- *Always use capsules.* Capsules break down more rapidly in the body, so you get to sleep more quickly. Capsules do not contain fillers or binders, so they are generally a purer product. The one exception is Mag Link; it cannot be encapsulated due to its chemical structure.

*Do not use if you are taking an SSRI, tricyclic, or MAO inhibitor antidepressant.
**Do not use if you have PKU, have had a melanoma, are pregnant or lactating, or if you use MAO inhibitors or tricyclic antidepressants.

- Play a relaxation tape to help you relax, and to promote sleep.
- Use deep-breathing exercises for 10 to 15 minutes, to relax the body and mind.
- Play some gentle, relaxing music an hour before you go to bed to allow your body to come down from your stressful day and prepare your body for sleep. Take a warm bath to relax your body for sleep.

Leaky Gut Syndrome

Leaky gut syndrome (LGS) is, simply, increased intestinal permeability. Someone with LGS exhibits many symptoms and illnesses. The precipitating causes of LGS include: abnormal flora (yeast, bacteria, parasites, etc.), food allergies, chemicals or drugs that irritate the small intestines or gut, chronic stress syndrome, and enzyme deficiencies, either genetic or acquired. At least 70% of our immune system is based on the health of our gut.

The digestive tract is vitally important for total body health. The intestinal tract, or gut, must be healthy, or the rest of the body suffers.

Symptoms Associated with LGS

- Abdominal pain
- Aggressive behavior
- Anxiety
- Asthma
- Bed-wetting
- Bladder infections, recurring
- Bloating
- Candida
- Chronic joint pains
- Confusion
- Constipation
- Diarrhea
- Exercise intolerance
- Fatigue
- Fever of unknown reason
- Gas, upper and lower
- Indigestion
- Immunity poor
- Learning disorders
- Memory poor
- Mood swings
- Nervousness
- Muscle pains
- PMS
- Recurring infections
- Shortness of breath
- Skin rashes
- Fuzzy or spacey thinking
- Vaginal infections
- Yeast infections

The digestive tract is a 25-to-30 foot-long hose that starts at the mouth and ends at the anus. The gut's function includes the digestion, into microscopic particles, of the food we eat, and absorption and conversion of these particles into energy. The intestine is responsible for absorbing vitamins and minerals into the bloodstream, detoxifying major chemicals in the body, and synthesizing antibodies and immunoglobulins that act as the first line of defense against infections. The intestine performs a dual function. As it allows nutrients into the bloodstream, it prevents large molecules, bacteria, other microbes, and toxins from entering. But the small intestinal mucosa has only a single-cell thickness.

A healthy gut lining allows properly digested proteins, fats, and carbohydrates to pass into the intestinal villi, or small finger-like folds in the intestinal wall, while keeping out bacteria, large undigested molecules, and toxins. The gut repairs and replaces itself every three to six days. Leaky gut syndrome allows substances to pass through the intestinal lining that normally do not. Alcohol, foods, medications, and stress compromise the intestinal lining. These substances irritate and inflame the intestinal wall, and they cause tiny tears. The small intestinal lining develops large, leaky spaces between the cells of the intestinal walls, infringing the intestinal barrier, and allowing in bacteria, viruses, toxins, and foods. When there is a disruption of the normal intestinal flora, bacteria and fungus (yeast) overgrowth occurs, and immune-system resistance decreases. Normal flora disruption and increased intestinal permeability occur after surgery, nutritional tube-feedings, trauma from burns, severe blood loss, and other physical trauma.

The liver is the main organ that converts toxins or harmful substances into by-products that are excreted. Toxins can overload the liver. An overloaded liver does not detoxify, and allows extra toxins to enter the bloodstream. A person with chemical and food sensitivities can develop autoimmune antibodies and more food and chemical sensitivities. You might assume the body is able to absorb more amino acids, vitamins, minerals, and nutrients, but, instead, your body absorbs less of these vital nutrients.

Antibiotics and nonsteroidal anti-inflammatory medications (NSAIDs) such as aspirin, Motrin (ibuprofen), and Aleve, cause LGS. Antibiotics do not discriminate; they kill both good and bad bacteria

Common Conditions Associated with Leaky Gut Syndrome

- Acne
- Aging
- AIDS
- Alcoholism
- Allergies
- Ankylosing spondylitis
- Arthritis
- Asthma
- Autism
- Burns
- Candida infections (intestinal dysbiosis)
- Celiac disease
- Chemical sensitivities
- Chemotherapy
- Chronic fatigue
- Crohn's disease
- Cystic fibrosis
- Eczema
- Environmental Illness (EI)
- Fibromyalgia
- Food allergies/sensitivities
- Hyperactivity
- Inflammatory bowel disease
- Intestinal infections
- Irritable bowel syndrome
- Liver dysfunction
- Lupus
- Malabsorption
- Malnutrition
- NSAIDs ingestion
- Pancreatic insufficiency
- Nutritional deficiencies
- Poor diet
- Psoriasis
- Reiter's Syndrome
- Rheumatoid arthritis
- Trauma
- Ulcerative colitis

in the body and gut. Since antibiotics change the balance of the intestine, fungi (yeast), viruses, parasites, and resistant bacteria colonize the gut. These microbes contribute to inflammation, irritation, and leaky gut syndrome.

Steroids are used for allergies, asthma, autoimmune diseases, and inflammation. Long-term use of steroid medications, such as prednisone and nasal sprays for allergies, depresses the immune system and encourages yeast infections in the gut.

Chronic stress also contributes to LGS by inhibiting the body's ability to heal or respond rapidly. Stress causes our bodies to secrete less DHEA, an adrenal hormone that possesses anti-aging and anti-stress properties.

Food sensitivities/allergies promote inflammation in the body, including the gut. LGS develops and allows food particles to enter the

Causes of Leaky Gut Syndrome

- Aging
- Antibiotics
- AIDS
- Candida
- Chemotherapy
- Chronic stress
- Chronic infections
- Environmental contamination

- Enzyme deficiencies
- Food allergies
- Gastrointestinal (GI) diseases
- Immune-system overload
- Overindulgence of alcohol
- Parasites
- Steroid medications
- Trauma

bloodstream. As foreign substances to the body, these food particles trigger an immune response. Ingestion of foods to which you are sensitive causes increased intestinal permeability. The insulted gut allows more food particles to pass into the circulation, and, as a result, you develop more food sensitivities as antibody responses.

If you have leaky gut syndrome, how do you get well? You must heal your gut; and you must be patient with yourself, as it will take time for your body to recover.

1) Remove the cause.
2) Restore good GI function by eating well, using a food-rotation diet if you have multiple allergies. If you know specifically the foods causing the problem, leave them out of your diet for at least four to six months, to allow the intestines to heal. Chew your food thoroughly and increase the fiber in your diet.
3) Eat a caveman diet. Eat fresh fruits and vegetables, nuts, seeds, and low-sugar foods.
4) Don't expect miracles from your body in one or two days. Be patient and persist, to help your body recover so you feel better and have a better quality of life.

Suggested Nutritional Support

Digestive Enzymes – Take 1 or 2 digestive enzymes, in capsule form, such as Super Digestaway, and 1 pancreatin capsule with each meal. The digestive enzymes help your body thoroughly digest ingested foods and to break down the foods into smaller particles, so they are less antigenic. Always make sure your digestive enzyme is in capsule form; tablets sometimes pass through your body without being absorbed.

Acidophilus – Take 1 or 2 acidophilus bifidus capsules, four times daily. Reintroduce some good intestinal flora into the gut or intestine. If you are not allergic to milk, you can also take a teaspoon of "live-cultured" yogurt, twice daily.

Super Glutamine – Take 1000 mg of Super Glutamine (pure pharmaceutical grade powder), three to four times daily, to help repair the small and large intestines. The GI tract, especially the small intestine, is the greatest user of glutamine in the body. Glutamine is vital for our health.

Deluxe Scavenger – Take 3 capsules daily, divided. Deluxe Scavengers contain a mixture of the antioxidants in one capsule. This combination formula comprises CoEnzyme Q10, beta-carotene, Vitamin C, lemon bioflavonoids, rutin, Vitamin E, selenium, glutathione, NAC, riboflavin, P5'P, and Vitamin B6.

T-L Vite – 1 capsule with the main meal of the day.

Anxiety Control 24 – 1 or 2 capsules, three to four times daily, for stress and anxiety.

Or Use Mood Sync* – 1 or 2 capsules, three times daily for stress with depression.

Ester C – 2,000 to 4,000 mg, per day, divided.

Garlic – 1,500 to 3,000 mg, per day, divided. Garlic helps maintain a healthy intestine, promoting the proper bacteria in the gut.

Alka-Seltzer Gold – Use 1 capsule as needed to neutralize a food reaction.

*Do not take if you are currently taking an SSRI or MAO inhibitor medication.

Menopausal Stress/Anxiety

Many women experience anxiety just before menopause. Your body is undergoing a major transition; you must be patient and allow your brain and body to adjust to all the changes. Using amino acids for stress and anxiety will lessen the fear and uncertainty.

Suggested Nutritional Support

T-L Vite – 1 capsule daily. T-L Vite is a multivitamin/mineral designed beneficial for postmenopausal women.

Mood Sync* – 1 or 2 capsules, twice to three times daily.

B Complex – 1 capsule, daily, in the morning with breakfast.

B.N.C. Plus GABA – 1 teaspoon in fruit juice in morning and the evening.

GABA 750 – 1/2 capsule in herbal tea or cup of water in the morning and mid afternoon.

5-HTP* – 1 or 2 capsules, 30 minutes prior to bedtime.

Liquid Serotonin – Use 10 to 15 drops, under the tongue, twice daily, and at bedtime.

Carnitine – 500 mg capsule twice daily, morning and afternoon.

Mag Link – 2 in the morning and 2 in the afternoon. If loose stools occur, decrease the dosage by one.

DHEA** – 1 capsule daily, (25 mg or 50 mg, depending on age) upon arising in morning.

Pregnenolone** – 1 to 2 (10 mg) capsule, daily.

Balanced Woman – 1 to 2 capsule(s), twice daily helps balance a women's circulatory and hormonal systems. Balanced Woman formula is a traditional Chinese medicine formula designed to promote optimal health by establishing the body's natural balance.

Dong Quai*** – 2 (1000 mg) capsules, twice to three times daily for perimenopausal stress. Dong Quai is an adaptogen that brings your body into balance. Dong Quai does not contain any estrogen or phytoestrogens or any type of estrogenic activity. Dong Quai contains mild sedative properties and brings on menstruation.

Soy – 1 to 2 servings per day of either powder form or capsules form with isoflavones. Soy provides phytoestrogens helping to replace estrogen that drops at menopause.

If you are stressed out or anxious prior to meals, use Liquid Serotonin 10 to 15 drops and ¼ capsule of GABA 750 dissolved in 8 ounces of warm water. Stress causes a release of insulin and adrenaline that tightens up the digestive muscles, causing bloating. If this is a chronic condition, consider digestive enzymes.

---

*Do not use if you are taking an SSRI, tricyclic, or MAO inhibitor antidepressant.

**For additional information on DHEA and dosing, read Health Educator Report #51, and for Pregnenolone, read Health Educator Report #20.

***Do not use if you are on antihypertensive or anticoagulant medications.

Obsessive-Compulsive Disorder (OCD)

Anxious thoughts, or rituals, that you feel you cannot control, characterize obsessive-compulsive disorder (OCD). Persistent, unwelcome thoughts or images, and the urgent need to engage in certain rituals can plague you, if you have OCD.

You may be obsessed with germs, or dirt, so you wash your hands over and over. You can be filled with doubt, and feel the need to check things again and again. You might be preoccupied by thoughts of violence, and fear that people close to you will be harmed. You may spend long periods of time touching things or counting. Order or symmetry may preoccupy you. You may be worried by thoughts that are against your religious beliefs.

These disturbing thoughts or images are called obsessions. The rituals performed to prevent or dispel them are called compulsions. There is no pleasure in carrying out the rituals that you are drawn to— only temporary relief from the discomfort caused by the obsession.

Many healthy people can identify with having some of the symptoms of OCD, such as checking the stove several times before leaving the house. But the disorder is usually diagnosed only when such activities consume at least an hour a day, prove very distressing, and interfere with daily life. Most adults with this condition recognize the senselessness of their condition, but they cannot stop. Although some people, especially children with OCD, may not realize their behavior is unusual. OCD strikes men and women in approximately equal numbers, and afflicts roughly 1 in 50 people. It can appear in childhood, adolescence, or adulthood, but usually starts in the teens or early adulthood. A third of adults with OCD experience their first symptoms as children. The course of the disease varies. Symptoms can come and go. They may ease over time, or they can grow progressively worse. Evidence suggests that OCD might run in families.

Depression or other anxiety disorders can accompany OCD. Some people with OCD have eating disorders. Additionally, they avoid situations in which they might have to confront their obsessions. They may try unsuccessfully to use alcohol or drugs to calm themselves. If the OCD grows severe enough, it can keep someone from holding down a job, or from carrying out normal responsibilities at home. Frequently, however, the disorder does not develop to those extremes.

Research by National Institutes of Mental Health scientists and other investigators led to the development of amino acid and behavioral treatments benefiting people with OCD. A combination of the treatments often benefits most patients. Some individuals respond best to one therapy, some to another. Behavioral therapy, specifically a type called *exposure and response prevention,* has also proven useful for treating OCD. It involves exposing the person to whatever triggers the problem, and then helping him or her forego the usual ritual. For instance, having the patient touch something dirty and then not washing his hands. This therapy succeeds in patients who complete a behavioral therapy program, although results have been less favorable in some people who have both OCD and depression. Address OCD and depression separately.

With OCD, as well as depression, research demonstrates that serotonin is involved in the biology of obsessive-compulsive behavior. As serotonin levels decrease, OCD behavior becomes more pervasive. Anxiety, depression, stress, especially post-traumatic stress disorder and grief, use available serotonin. Those who suffer from OCD are victims of a serotonin–dopamine interaction gone wrong. Both serotonin and dopamine are the primary neurotransmitters in the brain's frontal lobes, where decisions are made. Neurotransmitters are the chemical agents responsible for transmitting impulses between nerve fibers, or from nerve fibers to a specific receptor. Using a balanced neurotransmitter complex, on a daily basis, along with 5-HTP, helps balance serotonin and dopamine levels.

Suggested Nutritional Support

Brain Link Complex – 3 scoops dissolved in juice, first thing in the morning.

Or Use **TL-Vite** – 1 capsule, in the morning.

Glutamine – 1,000 mg, in either capsules or powder, three times per day.

B.N.C. Plus GABA – 1 teaspoon in fruit juice, mid morning, and mid afternoon or if you prefer capsules, use 3 BNC capsules in the morning and in the afternoon.

GABA 750 – ½ capsule dissolved in water, mid morning and mid afternoon.

Mood Sync* – 1 or 2 capsules, twice to three times daily. Mood Sync combines 5-HTP, St. John's Wort, GABA, glutamine, taurine, and B6.

Or Use **Tyrosine 850***– 1 in the morning, and 1 in the evening. If under 100 pounds, use tyrosine (500 mg), 1 in the morning and 1 in the evening. Do not take if you are taking an MAO inhibitor or tricyclic antidepressant.

Liquid Serotonin – 10 to 15 drops, four times per day, or as needed.

5-HTP** – 2 capsules, 1 hour before bedtime.

Mag Link – 1 to 2 tablet(s), three times per day, depending on weight. If loose stools or diarrhea occurs, decrease by 1 tablet, or try increasing the time between doses.

B Complex Capsule – 1 capsule in the morning.

Methionine – 500 mg in the morning, and in the evening.

*Do not use if you have PKU, have had a melanoma, are pregnant or lactating, or if you use MAO inhibitors or tricyclic antidepressants.

**Do not use if you are taking an SSRI, tricyclic, or MAO inhibitor antidepressant.

Panic Disorder

Panic disorder strikes at least 1.8% of the population, and is twice as common in women than in men. It can appear at any age, but most often it begins in young adults. Not everyone who experiences panic attacks will develop panic disorder. Many people have one attack, but never have another. If you do have panic disorder, it is important to seek treatment. If untreated, the disorder can become very disabling.

People with panic disorder experience sudden feelings of terror, repeatedly with no warning. While impossible to predict when an attack will occur, many develop intense anxiety between episodes, worrying when and where the next one will strike. In between times there is a persistent, lingering worry that another attack could come any minute.

When a panic attack strikes, your heart pounds and you feel sweaty, weak, faint, or dizzy. Your hands tingle or feel numb, and you feel flushed, or chilled. You can have chest pain or smothering sensations,

Panic Attack Symptoms

- Pounding heart
- Chest pains
- Light-headedness or dizziness
- Nausea or stomach problems
- Hot flushes or chills
- Tingling or numbness
- Shaking or trembling
- Feelings of unreality
- Shortness of breath
- Sensation of choking or smothering
- Tremors
- A feeling of being out of control or going crazy
- Fear of dying
- Sweating

a sense of unreality, fear of impending doom, or loss of control. You genuinely believe you are having a heart attack or stroke, losing your mind, or on the verge of death. Attacks can occur any time, even during non-dream sleep. While most attacks average a couple of minutes, occasionally they can go on for up to 20 minutes.

Often accompanied by other conditions such as depression or alcoholism, panic disorder may spawn phobias which can develop in places or situations where panic attacks have occurred. If a panic attack strikes while you are riding an elevator you can develop a fear of elevators, and start avoiding them.

Many people's lives become greatly restricted. You avoid normal, everyday activities such as grocery shopping, driving, or even leaving your home. You may be able to confront a feared situation only if accompanied by a spouse or other trusted person. Basically, you avoid any situation you fear might make youfeel helpless if a panic attack occurs. When a person's life becomes so restricted by the disorder, as happens in approximately one third of all people with panic disorder, the condition is called agoraphobia. A tendency toward panic disorder and agoraphobia runs in families. Often, early treatment of panic disorder can stop the progression to agoraphobia.

Studies have shown proper treatment called cognitive behavioral therapy, orthomolecular therapy, or a combination of the two, helps 70 to 90% of people with panic disorder. Significant improvement occurs within 8 to 10 days.

The cognitive behavioral approach teaches you how to view the panic situations differently, and demonstrates ways to reduce anxiety by using breathing exercises or techniques to refocus your attention. Another technique used in cognitive behavioral therapy is called exposure therapy. This frequently helps alleviate the phobias resulting from panic disorder. In exposure therapy, you are very slowly exposed to the fearful situation a number of times until you become desensitized.

Most people find the greatest relief from panic disorder symptoms when they use orthomolecular therapy. Orthomolecular and cognitive behavioral therapies, can help relieve panic attacks and reduce their frequency.

Suggested Nutritional Support

Panic and anxiety can cause feelings of fatigue and loss of appetite. Nutrients taken daily in the morning are readily absorbed and give you a needed lift.

Brain Link Complex – Take in 8 ounces of fruit juice, and follow directions on can (dosage depends on weight).

Anxiety Control 24 – 2 capsules, early morning, noon, and evening. Add 2 additional, if needed for panic.

Or Use **GABA 750** – ½ capsule dissolved in water, mid morning. Repeat mid afternoon and evening. If under 125 pounds, use GABA 375 dissolved in water.

Liquid Serotonin – 10 to 15 drops, three times per day.

Mag Link – 2 tablets, twice to three times daily. Titrate to bowel tolerance. If loose stool/diarrhea occurs, try spreading out further, or decrease by 1.

Taurine 1000 – 1 capsule, twice daily.

5-HTP* – 1 (50 mg), an hour before bedtime.

PoweRelief**– 2 capsules, as needed for pain.

*Do not use if you are taking an SSRI, tricyclic, or MAO inhibitor antidepressant.
**Do not use if you have PKU, have had a melanoma, are pregnant or lactating, or if you use MAO inhibitors or tricyclic antidepressants.

Premenstrual Syndrome (PMS)

Premenstrual Syndrome, or PMS, is a very distressing syndrome for many women. It commonly occurs in women of child-bearing age, 7 to 10 days prior to onset of her period. The degree varies, but at least 50% of all women experience at least some symptoms of PMS. PMS bothers some women from the onset of menses, but most commonly, it affects women in the thirties and into the perimenopausal years. In about half of these, the symptoms manifests so severely they need treatment or medical attention.

There are various risk factors for PMS. Advancing age and the number of children increase the development of PMS. As a woman ages, the more painful periods experienced by women in their teens and twenties are often replaced by the appearance of PMS symptoms. The most severe and difficult cases of PMS are usually found in women in their forties. PMS symptoms usually start to overlap menopausal symptoms.

Suggested Nutritional Support

Rodex B6 (timed-release) – 1 capsule (150 mg) in the morning.

Anxiety Control 24 – For irritability and anxiety, use 2, three times per day.

Mood Sync* – 1 or 2 capsules, twice to three times daily, as needed for mood swings and depression.

Categories of PMS Symptoms

PMS A   anxiety, nervous tension, mood swings, irritability

PMS B   weight gain, swelling of breasts and extremities, breast tenderness, abdominal bloating

PMS C   headache, increased appetite, cravings for sweets, fatigue, dizziness, fainting, pounding heart

PMS D   depression, forgetfulness, crying, confusion, and insomnia

Other   oily skin, acne, clumsiness, feelings of violence, or even suicide in severe cases

Tyrosine 850**– For depression, 1 in the morning and 1 mid afternoon.

Glycine – 1 or 2 capsules dissolved under tongue to cut sugar cravings.

Mag Link – 4 to 6 tablets per day, divided. Take to bowel tolerance, then decrease by one. Magnesium is extremely important for many symptoms of PMS, including anxiety, painful menstruation, and headache prior to period. Be patient with painful menstruation as it may take several months to increase your magnesium level.

PowerRelief** – For pain relief, use 1 or 2 capsules, as needed.

T-L Vite – 1 capsule daily with main meal. T-L Vites are a combination multivitamin/mineral.

Glutamine – For memory and concentration, use 1 (500 mg) capsule, or ½ scoop glutamine powder, three times per day.

Chromium Picolinate – For sugar cravings and to help stabilize blood sugar, use 1(200 mcg), twice per day.

5-HTP* – For sleep and to balance the serotonin level, take 1 (50 mg) capsule 30 minutes before bedtime.

Vitamin E – For breast tenderness, increase up to 2,000 I.U. a week before your period, then decrease and maintain with no more than 800 I.U. of vitamin E per day.

Progesterone Cream (such as ProgestaCare) – 1 pump or 20 mg applied to back of hand or forearm once daily, as needed. Progesterone improves your mood and increases libido. Progesterone counterbalances the toxic effects of estrogen dominance.

DHEA – 1 (25 mg) upon arising in the morning, if you are over 40 years of age.

Pregnenolone – 10 to 50 mg upon arising in the morning, if you are over 40 years of age.

- Avoid caffeine, colas, and sugar to decrease anxiety, insomnia, nervousness. Colas and caffeine cause a loss of magnesium which amplify stress and anxiety.
- Avoid coffee, chocolate, cola based sodas, and high intake of salt based foods, to decrease fluid retention and breast tenderness.
- Reduce tobacco intake.
- Reduce the intake of fats; avoid fried foods and animal fats.

*Do not use if you are taking an SSRI or MAO inhibitor drug.

**Tyrosine, Phenylalanine, or DLPA should not be taken by pregnant or lactating women, those with PKU, if you are taking MAO inhibitors or tricyclic antidepressants, or if you have had a malignant melanoma.

- Increase intake of fiber with complex carbohydrates, leafy vegetables, legumes, and fruits.
- Limit intake of alcohol, refined sugar, and red meat.
- Reduce stress through regular exercise. Use other stress-reduction techniques such as massage, meditation, and relaxation tapes.

Post Traumatic Stress Disorder (PTSD)

Patients demonstrate symptoms of generalized anxiety and reoccurring flashbacks of traumatic episodes. PTSD usually occurs after a severe major stressor: fire, tornado, major auto accident, unexpected death, or military experience. Weeks or months after the traumatic episode occurs, flashbacks can begin and cause numerous physical symptoms such as sweating, rapid pulse, increased anxiety, panic, insomnia, and avoidance behaviors. Flashbacks can also cause a release of adrenaline. This sets stress reaction into high gear. Stress burns amino acids, and unless the brain is supplied with nourishment, it will continue to send anxiety-related messages that cause physical symptoms. A therapist experienced in PTSD and a good orthomolecular program will be helpful and aid the healing process.

PTSD is a debilitating condition that affects thousands of people. Often, people with PTSD have persistent frightening thoughts and memories of their ordeal, and feel emotionally numb. PTSD was once referred to as shell shock, or battle fatigue. It was first brought to public attention by war veterans. But, it can result from any number of traumatic incidents, serious accidents, natural disasters such as floods or earthquakes, or violent attacks such as mugging, rape, kidnapping, or torture. The event triggering the post trauma may be something that threatened the person's life, or the life of someone close to them, or it can be something they witnessed, such as the Oklahoma City bombing.

People with PTSD can relive the trauma in the form of nightmares, or disturbing recollections in which they experience the event over and over in their minds. They may also experience sleep problems, depression, feelings of detachment or numbness, or be easily startled. They may lose interest in things they once enjoyed, and have trouble showing affection. Sometimes, they feel more irritable or more aggressive than before the incident, and can even become violent. Memories that remind them of the incident can be very distressing, causing them to avoid certain places or situations that bring back to the event. Even anniversaries of the event are often very difficult.

PTSD can happen at any age. The disorder can be accompanied by anxiety, depression, or substance abuse. Symptoms may be mild or severe. People may become easily irritated or have violent outbursts. In severe cases they may have trouble working or socializing. In general, the symptoms seem to be worse if the event that triggered them was initiated by a person, such as a mugging or rape, as opposed to something like a flood.

Ordinary events can serve as reminders of the trauma and trigger flashbacks or intrusive memories. A flashback may make the person lose touch with reality and reenact the event for a period of seconds or hours, rarely days. A person having a flashback, which can come in the form of images, sounds, smells, or feelings, believes the traumatic incident is happening all over again.

Not every traumatized person gets full-blown PTSD, some don't experience PTSD at all. If the symptoms last more than a month, PTSD is the diagnosis. Symptoms usually occur within 3 months of the trauma, but the course of the illness varies. Some people recover within 6 months; others have symptoms that last much longer. The condition can become chronic. In some cases, PTSD may not arise until years after the traumatic event.

Amino acids can ease the symptoms of depression and sleep problems, but psychotherapy, especially cognitive behavioral therapy, is an integral part of treatment. Being exposed to a reminder of the trauma as part of the therapy, such as returning to the scene, sometimes helps. Support from family and friends can help speed recovery.

Antidepressants and tranquilizers only postpone healing and suppress symptoms. They do not restore the brain chemistry with needed nutrients.

Suggested Nutritional Support

B.N.C. Plus GABA – 1 teaspoon in fruit juice, morning and evening.

Liquid Serotonin – 10 to 12 drops, 2 to 4 times daily, and if you awaken during the night.

Rodex B6 – 1 (150 mg timed release) capsule in the morning.

TL Vite (multivitamin) – 1 capsule, in the morning with breakfast.

Mag Link – 4 to 6 tablets per day, divided, throughout the day, up to bowel tolerance, then back decrease by one.

Anxiety Control 24 – 2 capsules, three times daily, for the first month after a traumatic episode, then 2 in the morning and 2 in the afternoon. Increase to 6 per day, if needed.

Ester C – 1,000 mg, morning and evening.

Powerelief*– 2 capsules (300 mg), twice daily, as needed for pain. As an alternative, use Mobigesic, boswella, or DLPA.

Mood Sync**– If depression occurs, take 2 capsules, twice daily.

5-HTP** – 1 (50 mg) at bedtime. Take 2, if your sleep pattern is interrupted.

Or Use **Melatonin** – For sleep use 3 mg, an hour before bedtime.

- Do not use alcohol in the acute stage of trauma.
- Decrease caffeine intake, and have none after noon.
- Limit sugar and soda intake.
- During the first month, avoid loud noises and bright lights.
- Use relaxation tapes, two to three times per week.

*Do not use if you have PKU, have had a melanoma, are pregnant or lactating, or if you use MAO inhibitors or tricyclic antidepressants.

**Do not use if you are taking an SSRI, tricyclic, or MAO inhibitor antidepressant.

Post-Trauma Case History

Kelly is a 36-year old college professor who never had any major problems with anxiety or chronic pain until May 15, 1994. That day, while driving to the University, Kelly's life took a turn for the worse. She was hit broadside by a teenager. Her car was totaled, and so was her life.

Kelly spent a week in the hospital for painful neck and back injuries. Her healing was slow, and she had to learn to live with chronic pain and certain restrictions. But each day, Kelly improved a little more and tried to put her life back in order.

A few months passed without any particular problems. Then one day while driving to her classes, she heard a sound that she had hoped she would never hear again ... A car, unable to stop, slammed into the car in front of her. Kelly was not hurt, but she was so full of fear she had a full-blown panic attack. This was the beginning of her post-traumatic stress disorder, and all the symptoms that go with it. As time went on, she began having flashbacks of her accident, and with the flashbacks came the physical symptoms. Kelly developed a dread of driving because she never knew when the flashbacks would occur. Her physical symptoms included palpitations, weakness, trembling, apprehensiveness, sweating, headaches, muscle spasms, and fear of dying. Kelly came in to see me. I explained post-traumatic stress disorder and the symptoms. I started her on a relaxation program and nutritional supplements. She was totally depleted of neurotransmitters because of the chronic stress. Kelly's nutritional support program included Anxiety Control, Mag Link, Powerelief, and B-complex. Within a few weeks she showed a marked improvement. Her headaches stopped, and her driving anxiety diminished. Post-traumatic stress disorder can cause numerous psychological and physical problems, but with proper therapy, healing will occur.

Drugs that Deplete Melatonin

NSAIDs (Non-Steroidal Anti-Inflammatory Drugs) such as aspirin, ibuprofen (Motrin), Lodeine, Orudis, Aleve, Dolobid.
Tranquilizers such as Valium, Ativan.
Anti-anxiety meds such as Xanax, Ativan, Prozac.
Calcium channel blockers such as Cardizem, Procardia, Verapamil.
Beta blockers such as Inderal, Lopressor, Tenormin.
Steroids such as hydrocortisone, prednisone, Depo-Medrol.
Antidepressants such as Prozac, Serzone, Effexor, Luvox.
Vitamin B12 in large doses.

Source: Dr. Russel J. Reiter, University of Texas Health Science Center in San Antonio

Seasonal Affective Disorder (SAD)

Seasonal Affective Disorder, or SAD, is the only illness that demonstrates evidence of circadian rhythm disturbances. The symptoms of SAD occur only on a seasonal basis. Classical depression exhibits a daily rhythm that worsens in the morning and improves in the evening, with mood swings, and insomnia or disturbed sleep patterns. SAD symptoms always begin in autumn or early winter. SAD usually lasts five to seven months, until spring, when the days grow considerably longer, and the symptoms disappear. The person remains healthy until the following fall. Incidences of SAD increase almost proportionately to how far people live from the equator.

Four classic symptoms occur every fall and winter in most SAD sufferers:

- Increased desire to sleep
- Extreme lethargy
- Depression
- Increased appetite (which often leads to weight gain)

Melatonin greatly benefits SAD sufferers. Depression and melancholy are linked to a deficiency of neurotransmitters and neurohormones. Melatonin, taken nightly, supports the delicate brain balance.

The disruption of circadian rhythms can lead to stress-induced immunosuppression. Melatonin serves as an important anti-stress buffer. People with free-floating anxiety—anxiety without apparent cause—phobias, insomnia, and depression tend to have lower than normal levels of melatonin. Many of their

---

Direct Circadian Rhythm Influencers

- Sleep/wake cycle.
- Neurotransmitters/neuropeptides.
- Hormones.
- Other factors such as age, mood changes, body temperature, blood pressure and pulse rate, jet lag.

symptoms ease after supplementing with melatonin. People with anxiety report marked improvement after adding melatonin and other inhibitory neurotransmitters.

Suggested Nutritional Support

Melatonin – 2 mg capsule, 30 minutes before bedtime. If you weigh over 200 pounds, use 3 mg. Melatonin regulates the circadian rhythm.

DHEA – 1 (25 mg) capsule, first thing in the morning, on an empty stomach, if you are over 40. DHEA helps stressed adrenals.

Mood Sync* – 1 or 2 capsules, twice daily, for stress and anxiety with depression. St. John's Wort lowers the amount of light needed to obtain therapeutic effect.

Or Use **HTP10***– 2 capsules, twice daily.

Or Use **5-HTP*** – 1 (50-mg) capsule in the morning. 5-HTP is a direct precursor to serotonin, and it elevates your mood. 5-HTP is present in Mood Sync and HTP10.

Ginkgo – 40 mg, every morning. Ginkgo prevents metabolic and neural disturbances, and increases blood flow to the brain.

Ginseng – 1 capsule, twice daily, for adaptogenic influence on energy.

*Do not use if you are taking an SSRI, tricyclic, or MAO inhibitor antidepressant.

Everything that happens in your brain—every thought, every memory, and every will to move a muscle— happens because of the release of neurotransmitters.

Teen Anger and Aggression
Neurotransmitter Deficiency

What makes some teenagers display angry and aggressive behavior, while others are calm and in control?

A growing number of scientists are looking at the delicate limbic system—the same area of the brain involved in ADD and ADHD. Research demonstrates alterations of function in the limbic system can cause changes in emotional responses like rage, fear, reasoning, and impulse control. The limbic system connects key parts of the brain such as the amygdala, hippocampus, and the cerebral cortex. All memories begin in the hippocampus, and all memories are stored in the amygdala. The limbic system marks all negative experiences for playback at a later time, especially experiences such as being abused as a child, or exposure to violent behavior.

The environmental factor of growing up in a dysfunctional home causes teens to demonstrate aggressive behavior. But the majority of evidence gathered about aggressive behavior points to disturbed brain function and the overproduction of certain chemicals and the under production of others. Studies done at the University of Illinois Medical School found children and teens, with aggressive and disruptive behavior, all had low levels of the major inhibitory neurotransmitter serotonin. Serotonin levels most accurately predict how teens and children will react to punishment. Serotonin transmits electrical impulses in the brain from one neuron to another. Low levels of serotonin interrupt the smooth transmission of impulses, and the brain receives mixed signals. According to Ronald Kotulak, author of *Inside the Brain*, scientists now believe that, along with the nation's increase in violence, low serotonin may be responsible for a steady increase in depression, especially among children.

Blood tests done on one hundred teens and children at the Pain & Stress Center all reflected major deficiencies of neurotransmitters. When the deficiencies were corrected with amino acid supplementation, behavior problems ranging from aggression, anger, ADD, ADHD, behavioral disorders, poor concentration, and depression, all diminished remarkably. Inborn metabolic errors,

Deficiency Symptoms of Low Serotonin in Teens and Adults

- Aggression
- Depression
- Anxiety
- Panic attacks
- Mood swings
- Violent tendencies
- Hyperactivity
- Migraine headaches
- PMS Syndrome
- Carbohydrate cravings
- Insomnia
- Obesity
- Fibromyalgia
- Alcoholism
- Obsessive-compulsive behavior
- Chronic pain

chronic stress and anxiety, as well as overconsumption of junk food, caffeine, sugar, and alcohol, can cause neurotransmitter deficiencies. And chronic stress burnout can kill brain cells.

Scientists have also reported a tendency for aggression can be inherited and found in aggressive genes. This predisposes a teen to anger, violence, and depression, and this gene could be passed on to his or her children. Children who have an alcoholic parent can inherit the alcoholic gene, and demonstrate the same amino acid deficiencies that cause the craving for alcohol. GABA and glutamine, two major neurotransmitters, shut off the craving switch in the brain. When the brain chemistry is in balance, impulsive and aggressive behavior patterns do not dominate brain function.

Serotonin enables impulses in the brain to harmonize. Serotonin-producing cells send out over five hundred thousand connections to cells in every part of the brain. Serotonin is the only neurotransmitter able to do that. For teens, the best serotonin source is 5-HTP, or 5-Hydroxytryptophan. The formula, Teen Link, is specially formulated for the teen's brain. Teen Link contains 5-HTP, GABA, Glutamine, St. John's Wort, Taurine, and B6.

There is no one solution to teen anger and violence. In addition to supplementing children's diets with amino acids, parents should consider counseling sessions with a behavior therapist for their children. Behavior therapists are trained in talk therapy and can help troubled teens sort out their feelings, and feel better about themselves. The longer negative feelings stay buried, the more powerful they become. This brain activity not only uses all available neurotransmitters, it also sets up a chain reaction that causes a teen to withdraw and allow his or her problems to go unresolved.

Drugs do not create new and needed neurotransmitters. Parents mistakenly put their children on Prozac, Zoloft, Serzone, or other drugs, to elevate their children's serotonin levels. These drugs only *use* available neurotransmitters. *Drugs do not create new needed neurotransmitters.* Drugs only mask symptoms and repress anger that should be resolved. There are neurotransmitter formulas available that can be given to children and teens safely, without the possibility of addiction or side effects.

The brain produces the only chemicals you will ever need. The key is to correct neurotransmitter imbalances in the brain and control aggression by adjusting brain levels of serotonin. Available serotonin declines in situations where chronic stress controls a person's life. Impulsive and angry behavior becomes a way of life, setting the stage for possible violent behavior. The teen's brain never slows down, and must be provided on a daily basis with proper nourishment in the form of balanced neurotransmitters. A complete neurotransmitter formula should contain the amino acids phenylalanine, leucine, valine, histidine, arginine, lysine, isoleucine, alanine, glutamine, methionine, threonine, alpha-ketoglutaric acid (Alpha KG), plus B6 and chromium that act as activating agents.

Suggested Nutritional Support

T-L Vite – 1 capsule with main meal. T-L Vite is a high quality multivitamin/mineral.

Or Use Brain Link Complex – 2 scoops in the morning in fruit juice.

BNC (Balanced Neurotransmitter Complex) – 2 capsule in the morning; if over 150 pounds, use 3 capsules.

Mag Link – 1 tablet in the morning, afternoon, and evening.

Lysine – 1 capsule (500 mg), twice to three times daily for facial or body skin problem, or herpes.

Anxiety Control 24 – 1 or 2 capsules, twice to three times daily for stress and anxiety.

Teen Link* – 1 capsules in the morning, and in the afternoon. If over 125 pounds, use 2 capsules.

Cal Mag Zinc – 2 capsules, at bedtime. If over 150 pounds, use 3 capsules.

5-HTP* – 1 capsule (50 mg) at bedtime.

Or Use **Sedaplus,** if taking an SSRI medication.

*Do not use if you are taking an SSRI, tricyclic, or MAO inhibitor antidepressant.

Tourette's Syndrome

In the 1960s, the medical profession recognized Tourette's Syndrome to be among the most-pervasive movement disorders. Over the years, more cases were studied and clinical researchers began to accumulate results of studies from large groups of clients. Agreement was reached that the base symptoms of multiple motor and vocal tics were onset in childhood.

Over the past five to ten years, many changes occurred in the diagnosis and understanding of Tourette's Syndrome. The most significant is the relationship of Tourette's Syndrome to other tic disorders. Continued research demonstrated the association of behavior problems, especially attention deficit disorder, hyperactivity, and obsessive-compulsive disorder.

The clinical criteria for Tourette's Syndrome include the presence of multiple motor tics, vocal tics, and behavioral problems, as well as environmental context. The onset of Tourette's occurs between the ages of two and thirteen, and can intermittently worsen, especially during times of high stress, emotional tension, or stimulant use.

Simple motor tics are abrupt, brief, isolated movements such as eye blinks, head twitches, shoulder shrugs, or facial grimaces. The vocal tics include a variety of inarticulate noises and sounds, such as throat clearing, sniffing, grunting, and groaning. Tics may manifest themselves by virtually any body movement, noise, or certain nutrient deficiencies. According to Roger Kurlan, M.D., Department of Neurology, University of Rochester School of Medicine, some problems found in school-age children with Tourette's Syndrome include:

- Motor tics, phone tics, and mental energy expended in suppressing tics
- Obsessive-Compulsive behaviors
- Attention Deficit Disorder with hyperactivity
- School and other phobias, test anxiety, conduct disorder, or depression
- Short temper or argumentative
- Associated learning disabilities
- Poor social skills
- Low self-esteem
- Medication side effects

Gerald Golden, M.D., Director, Child Development Center and Professor of Pediatrics, Department of Neurology, University of Texas, published a paper in the *Psychiatric Annals,* July 1988, on the relationship between stimulant medication and tics. Dr. Golden states "all of the stimulant drugs commonly used to treat attention deficit disorder have been reported to increase tic response. Tourette's was precipitated by treatment with Ritalin, Dexedrine, and Cylert. Similar response has been reported with the use of Imipramine." His report reflects clinical evidence that supports the observation that stimulant drugs increase the severity of tics 25 to 50% in patients with Tourette's, and occasionally can precipitate Tourette's Syndrome in a patient who did not previously manifest symptoms of this disorder. Researchers concluded that obsessive-compulsive disorder can coexist with Tourette's Syndrome. It now appears that there is a genetic link for those with OCD and Tourette's Syndrome. If the family already has a history of multiple chemical sensitivities, the potential for children to display the symptoms increases. Sherry Rogers, M.D., author of *Tired or Toxic?*, reports the tics of Tourette's Syndrome represent abnormal "firings" of the nervous system. According to Dr. Rogers, the study of Tourette's Syndrome individuals can represent the entire field of environmental medicine and nutritional biochemistry. Some common mineral abnormalities, such as magnesium deficiency, can exist. Many individuals can have hidden food sensitivities, and dust, inhalants, and mold sensitivities. In her book, Dr. Rogers addresses the possibilities of environmental factors first, and then proceeds with a treatment program which has proven very successful. All the research points to evidence that Tourette's Syndrome can have multiple triggers, and those who present with the symptoms should be evaluated to establish the underlying causes. Patients treated with prescription medication(s) do not improve, and side effects from the medication can aggravate the symptoms and increase depression and a feeling of hopelessness.

Doris Rapp, M.D., author of *Is This Your Child's World?*, feels physicians should explore all aspects to determine the primary cause of Tourette's Syndrome, and that prescription drugs are certainly not the answer. Dr. Rapp suggests starting by using a process of eliminating toxic chemicals from the diet and environment: caffeine, foods, dust, molds and pollens. Exposure to certain chemicals such as gas, paint, or pesticides, can cause Tourette's Syndrome symptoms to become more overt. What is important is for parents to recognize what triggers Tourette's Syndrome symptoms in the first place. Caution should be taken by those who have Tourette's Syndrome to avoid commonly suspected triggers such as cigarette smoke, pesticides, perfumed products, animal hair, alcohol, dust, and areas with high-mold counts. After eliminating exposure to these chemicals, you will notice positive behavior changes and increased motor skills in people with Tourette's.

Suggested Nutritional Support
Brain Link – Add to your favorite fruit juice, according to weight. Brain Link Complex is a total neurotransmitter complex, in powder

form, for children; or for adults, if you prefer a drink formula. If you prefer a capsule, use 1 T-L Vite, along with 2 BNC (Balanced Neurotransmitter Complex) capsules. Teens can use either the Brain Link or the T-L Vite, plus the BNC caps.

Folic Acid – Add 1 (400 mcg) daily. Folic acid is important for neurological functioning.

Ester C – Children under 100 pounds, use 1,000 mg, daily. Adults use 1,000 mg, three times daily.

Mag Link – 1 to 3 tablets in divided doses, daily if over 100 pounds, *Or Use* Magnesium Chloride liquid, 1 teaspoon in fruit juice, every morning and evening. For children, use **Calcium Magnesium Liquid**. It has a peppermint taste. Follow the instructions on the bottle.

Anxiety Control – 1 or 2 capsules, as needed, to reduce stress and anxiety. Teens use 1 or 2 Teen Link. Children under 50 pounds, use an extra scoop of Brain Link.

Vitamin E – Adults use 800 I.U. of Vitamin E; teens and children use only 400 I.U.; if a child weighs less than 50 pounds, use 200 I.U. Use Vitamin E to improve symptoms of neurological dysfunction.

Serotonin Liquid – ½ dropper; use as needed, daily, for children and adults.

5-HTP* – 1 (50 mg) capsule, 30 minutes before bed. If sleep problems persist, use 2 capsules. Teens, use 1 5-HTP capsule (50 mg), *OR* 1 to 3 **HTP10** capsules. Children, use 1 to 2 HTP10 capsules, 30 minutes prior to bedtime.

Taurine – 1 (1000 mg) capsule, three times daily. For children, use 500 mg, three times daily.

Ginkgo Biloba – 1 (40 mg) capsule in the morning, in adults, or if over 100 pounds.

HTP10* – Children with Tourette's, ADD/ADHD, need additional neurotransmitters for school. HTP10 is a low-dose 5-HTP for children, or small adults. Use 1 HTP10 in the morning, and 1 after lunch, to help children stay on task and focus, or for excessive movement.

*Do not use if you are taking an SSRI, tricyclic, or MAO inhibitor antidepressant.

Amino Acid Testing

The body constantly conducts many complicated series of chemical reactions in precisely controlled ways to keep us healthy. Over 5,000 reactions occur every second in a cell. By utilizing the natural substances in optimal quantities to reestablish a normal balance, you can help correct the cause of some disease processes in a nontoxic way.

Amino acid metabolism disorders are becoming recognized as a major factor in many disease processes. Amino acid analysis is an analytical technique on the leading edge of nutritional biochemical medicine. It gives a new approach toward illness, and assists patients who have not responded to treatment as expected, or who present complex cases with diverse symptoms.

Amino acid analysis of urine or plasma goes a long way toward assessing vitamin and mineral status. Amino acid analysis measures the levels of amino acids in the body that affect many important processes. Additionally, it provides insights into the patient's functional needs for a wide variety of vitamins and minerals. Many of the enzymes which catalyze the interconversion of amino acids require vitamin and mineral cofactors to function optimally. In many cases where incomplete conversion of one product to another is due to sluggish enzymes, this indicates a functional need for increasing levels of a cofactor.

Amino Acid Analysis has proven helpful in treating:

- Chronic fatigue
- Candida infections
- Food and chemical sensitivities
- Immune system disorders
- Anxiety
- Depression
- Learning disorders
- ADD/Hyperactivity
- Behavioral disorders
- Eating disorders
- Cancer
- Hypoglycemia
- Diabetes
- Cardiovascular disease
- Seizures
- Headaches
- Arthritis
- Chronic pain

For detailed information, write or call the Pain & Stress Clinic at (210) 614-7246 Monday through Friday.

General Summary of Amino Acids

In order to absorb and assimilate *any amino acid,* you must take B6 or P5'P daily. The other important cofactor is magnesium. Magnesium is a facilitator, and is involved in over 300 enzyme reactions in the body.

ALANINE
• May be used as a source for the production of glucose.

Therapeutic dosages: 200 to 600 mg per day.

ARGININE
• Helpful in treatment of burns, elevated ammonia levels, and cirrhosis of the liver by detoxifying ammonia.
• Stimulates immune response by enhancing the production of T cells.
• Induces growth hormone release from the pituitary gland.
• Should be used with caution in schizophrenia.
• Intake should be kept low in herpes simplex and Epstein Barr virus interactions.
• Required for normal sperm count.
• Essential amino acid for children, not adults.
• Enhances fat metabolism.

Therapeutic dosages: Up to 3000 mg per day.

ASPARTIC ACID
• Protective function over the liver.
• Promotes mineral uptake in intestinal tract.
• Helps in ammonia detoxification.
• Acts to transport magnesium and potassium to the cells.

CARNITINE
- Helpful in clearing blood of triglycerides.
- Helpful in lowering cholesterol, and increasing HDL levels.
- Essential in transportation of long chain fatty acids into the cells where fats are converted into energy.
- In heart patients, increases exercise endurance.
- Increases muscle strength.
- In uremia or kidney disease, may reduce risk factor for athero-sclerosis and coronary heart disease.
- Helpful with depression.

Therapeutic dosages: 1000 to 3000 mg per day.

CITRULLINE
- Produces the amino acids, Arginine and Ornithine.
- Detoxifies ammonia or other "nitrogen" waste products.
- Stimulates growth hormone production.

CYSTEINE
- Derived from serine and methionine in the liver.
- A major sulfur containing amino acid.
- Helps maintain skin flexibility and texture by slowing abnormal cross linking of collagen.
- Helpful in prevention of free radical formation, an antioxidant.
- Useful in iron deficiency, anemia and promotion of iron absorption.
- Promotes red and white blood cell reproduction and tissue restoration in lung diseases.
- Provides strength of the hair (over 10% of hair is cysteine).
- Converts to cystine in lack of Vitamin C.
- Heavy metal chelator.
- Helps protect against effects of alcohol and pollution.
- Assists in prevention of cataracts.
- A derivative called NAC is helpful with asthma, bronchitis and sinus drainage by liquefying and thinning mucus.

- NAC helps in preventing side effects from chemo and radiation therapies.

Use with caution in diabetic, due to changes in insulin cycle.

Therapeutic dosages: 250 to 500 mg twice per day, divided.

CYSTINE
- Helpful with psoriasis and eczema.
- Enhances tissue recovery after surgery.
- Part of insulin molecule.
- High content in hair.
- Use with caution in people predisposed to stone formation in the liver or kidneys.

GABA (Gamma Amino Butyric Acid)
- Reduces anxiety/stress by decreasing limbic firing.
- Helps decrease muscular tension due to stress.
- Assists with hyperactivity and ADD.
- Crosses blood-brain-barrier.

Therapeutic dosages: 600 to 3000 mg per day, divided.

GLUTAMIC ACID
- Precursor of GABA.
- Component of glucose tolerance factor.
- Helpful with muscular dystrophy.
- Useful in maintaining the body's nitrogen balance.

GLUTAMINE
- Helpful in ulcer and intestinal healing.
- Helps protect body from effects of alcohol.
- Assists in treatment of alcoholism by decreasing the desire to drink.
- Crosses blood-brain-barrier.
- Aids mental functions such as memory and concentration.
- Helps reduce intestinal permeability with food allergies.

- Needed for production of other nonessential amino acids.
- Enhances effectiveness of chemotherapy and radiation treatments for cancer, while reducing toxicity and damage to the body.

Therapeutic dosages: 500 to 4000 mg per day, divided.

GLUTATHIONE
- Contains cysteine, glycine, glutamate.
- Helps reduce free radical formation.
- Neutralizes atmospheric substances such as petrochemicals and chlorine.
- Protective effect against radiation therapy.
- Transports other amino acids into the cell.

Therapeutic dosages: 1000 to 3000 mg per day, divided.

GLYCINE
- Simplest amino acid.
- Has sweet taste and readily dissolves in liquids.
- Inhibitory neurotransmitter.
- Helpful with anxiety and hyperactivity.
- Helps to remove lead from the body.
- Assists with epilepsy.
- Low levels reported in ALS.

Therapeutic dosages: 500 to 3000 mg per day, divided.

HISTIDINE
- Essential amino acids for infants, not adults.
- Helps relieve pain due to rheumatoid arthritis.
- Should always be taken with Vitamin C (Ester C).
- Use with caution in females prone to depression due to P.M.S.
- Mild anti-inflammatory effect.
- Metabolized into the neurotransmitter histamine, which is involved in smooth muscle function in blood vessels.
- Helps maintain the myelin sheath or insulator of certain nerves.

- Necessary for proper functioning of auditory nerves.
- Chelates toxic metals from the body.
- Helpful with nausea during pregnancy.

Therapeutic dosages: 1000 to 6000 mg per day.

ISOLEUCINE

- One of the Branche Chain Amino Acids, and should be taken as a group.

Therapeutic dosages: 250 to 700 mg per day. Best as BCAA group supplement.

LEUCINE

- Second of the Branched Chain Amino Acids, and should be taken as a group.
- Great producer of energy under many kinds of stress from trauma to surgery, infection, muscle training, and weight lifting.
- Only amino acid that can substitute for glucose while fasting.
- Stimulates insulin release which stimulates protein synthesis and inhibits protein breakdown.
- Helpful with Parkinson's disease in large doses.
- Use with all stress.

Therapeutic dosages: BCAA as a group, use 175 to 1200 mg per day.

LYSINE

- Found in muscle, connective and collagen tissues.
- Inhibits growth and replication of herpes and Epstein Barr viruses.
- Promotes growth, especially bone growth in infants and children, both requiring much larger amounts in an adults.
- Required for antibody formation.
- Tends to be low in vegetarians.

Therapeutic dosages: 1000 to 3000 mg per day with Vitamin C, divided.

METHIONINE
- One of the sulfur amino acids.
- Powerful antioxidant and detoxifies the liver.
- Gives rise to taurine.
- Helps to detoxify heavy metals from the body and excessive levels of histamine.
- Involved in synthesis of choline and adrenaline, lecithin, and Vitamin B12.
- Always take with B6 to inhibit synthesis of homocysteine which promotes plague deposits in arteries.
- Necessary so selenium is available to the body.

Therapeutic dosages: 800 to 3000 mg per day, divided.

ORNITHINE
- May reduce fat and increase muscle mass.
- Powerful stimulator of growth hormone production by pituitary gland.
- Assists in detoxification of ammonia in urea cycle.
- Stimulates immune system and enhances wound healing.
- May be useful in autoimmune disease such as arthritis.
- Can be converted in body to arginine, glutamine, or proline.
- Doses of 1000 mg in some people may cause insomnia.

Therapeutic dosages: 500 to 3000 mg per day, divided.

PHENYLALANINE
- A precursor of the catecholamines, epinephrine, norepinephrine, dopamine and dopa.
- May be helpful with appetite control by stimulating CCK (choleocephtokinin enzyme).
- Increases blood pressure in hypotension.

Note: Should not be taken with MAO and tricyclic antidepressants,

Phenylalanine → Tyrosine → Dopamine → Norepinephrine

Epinephrine

and when cancerous melanoma is present.

Therapeutic dosages: 500 to 2000 mg per day, divided.

PROLINE

- Helpful in lowering blood pressure.
- Important in muscle, tendon and collagen repairs.
- Assists in skin flexibility in relation to aging and sun exposure, and essential for skin health.
- A major amino acid in collagen if Vitamin C is present.

Therapeutic dosages: 500 to 1000 mg per day with Vitamin C.

TAURINE

- Manufactured in the body from methionine or cysteine in the liver with B6. Some zinc must be present in body for taurine to function properly.
- Found in foods of animal origin and one of the sulfur amino acids.
- Predominant amino acid found in heart and assists in balancing calcium and potassium in the heart.
- Under stress, more taurine is used in the body.
- Useful in Congestive Heart Failure patients by easing their physical signs and symptoms without side effects.
- Increases left ventricular heart performance without changes in blood pressure.
- Associated with retinal (eye) degeneration.
- Helpful with seizures and epilepsy.
- Detoxifier of secondary bile acids and toxins.
- Protects cell membranes.
- Frequently considered a neuromodulator.
- Zinc enhances taurine's effect.
- Helps decrease pain in chronic pain sufferers.

Therapeutic dosages: 500 to 3000 mg per day, divided.

THREONINE

- An essential amino acid which rises three times normal during pregnancy.

- Necessary for digestive and intestinal function.
- Prevents accumulation of fat in liver.
- Increases glycine levels in brain, and notably reduces ALS symptoms.
- Essential for mental health.

Therapeutic dosages: 100 to 500 mg per day.

TRYPTOPHAN (5-HTP or 5-hydroxytryptophan)

- An essential amino acid and neurotransmitter.
- Neurohormone found in organs throughout the body.
- Precursor of serotonin in brain.
- Precursor niacin, and effective in treating pellagra.
- Appears to assist in blood clotting mechanisms.
- Helpful with insomnia in doses of 500 to 2000 mg.
- Helpful in depression and schizophrenia.
- Useful in weight control.
- Helps with pain by elevating the pain threshold.
- Acts as mood stabilizer, calming aggression, obsessive behavior.
- Take with B6 with carbohydrates such as fruit juice for maximum uptake to brain.
- Has helped decrease tremors in Parkinson's patients.
- Currently unavailable in U.S. due to F.D.A.

Note: Should not be taken with SSRIs (Selective Serotonin Reuptake Inhibitors) drugs such as Prozac, Paxil, Luvox, or Effexor.

Therapeutic dosages: 5-HTP 50 to 100 mg day divided.

Tryptophan → 5-HTP → Serotonin

5-HTP is about 10 times stronger than tryptophan, and is only 1 step biochemically away from serotonin.

Normal tryptophan dose is 500 to 4000 mg per day, divided.

TYROSINE
* Useful in people with Parkinson's disease.
* Precursor to catecholamines, epinephrine, norepinephrine, dopamine and dopa.
* Precursor of thyroid hormones.
* Assists in normal brain function and supplier of neurotransmitters.
* Can be used in place of many antidepressants.
* Helps stabilize blood pressure.
* Involved in tissue pigmentation.
* Often called the *Stress* amino acid.

Note: Should not be taken with MAO and tricyclic antidepressants, and when cancerous melanoma is present.

Therapeutic dosages: 500 to 2000 mg per day, divided.

VALINE
* Third of the Branched Chain Amino Acids, and should be taken as a group, and an essential amino acid needed for the nitrogen balance in the body.
* Necessary for muscle coordination, mental and neural function.
* Helpful with inflammation.

Therapeutic Dosage: up to 1000 mg daily. Best if taken as BCAA.

Research from UCLA demonstrates if the brain of a fifty year old person could be fully emptied of all impression and memories it has stored and recorded on tape, the length of the tape would reach to the moon and back several times.

Food Sources of Some Amino Acids
(In descending order of concentration)

Arginine: poultry, meats, fish, beans, grains, nuts and seeds, gelatin, cereals (especially buckwheat, oatmeal, and millet), milk, cheese, eggs, wheat germ, vegetables (especially green peas, asparagus, broccoli, swiss chard, corn, potatoes, onion, spinach), avocados, chocolate.

Cysteine: meat, chicken, turkey, fish, grains, beans (especially soy), eggs, nuts, seeds, milk, cheese, cereals, couscous wheat.

Histidine: meats, chicken, turkey, fish, beans (especially soy), cheese, milk, eggs, grains, nuts, seeds, cereals, potatoes.

Isoleucine: chicken, turkey, meats, fish, beans (especially soy), milk, cheese, eggs, grains, cereals (especially millet), nuts, seeds, vegetables including swiss chard, corn, green peas, potatoes, spinach) avocado.

Leucine: chicken, turkey, fish, beans, milk, meats, cheese, eggs, grains, cereals (especially millet), nuts, seeds, gelatin, vegetables including sweet potatoes, potatoes, spinach, corn, green peas, asparagus, broccoli, swiss chard, mushrooms, tomatoes, avocado, wheat germ.

Lysine: chicken, turkey, meats, beans, dairy including milk, cheese, eggs, grains, cereals (especially oatmeal), gelatin, vegetables including potatoes, green peas, asparagus, broccoli, corn, mushrooms, spinach, avocado, wheat germ, chocolate.

Methionine: chicken, poultry, meats, fish, grains, beans, nuts, seeds, cereals (especially couscous, millet, and oatmeal), gelatin.

Phenylalanine: chicken, turkey, meats, fish, dairy including milk, cheese; eggs, beans, grains, cereals (especially millet and oatmeal), nuts, seeds, vegetables including sweet potatoes, potatoes, spinach, corn, green peas, swiss chard, gelatin, avocado, chocolate.

Threonine: chicken, turkey, meats, fish, beans, dairy including milk, cheese; eggs, grains, nuts, seeds, cereals, gelatin, some vegetables including corn, green peas, potatoes, and spinach.

Trytophan: turkey, chicken, pork, meats, fish, beans, dairy including milk, cheese; eggs, grains, cereals, nuts, seeds.

Tyrosine: chicken, turkey, pork, beef, fish, beans, dairy including milk, cheese; cereals (especially oatmeal and couscous), some vegetables including corn, potatoes, spinach, nuts, seeds.

Valine: chicken, turkey, pork, beef, fish, dairy including milk, cheese; cereals (especially millet, buckwheat groats, oatmeal); some vegetables including potatoes, sweet potatoes, broccoli, corn, green peas, spinach, swiss chard; avocado, and chocolate.

Source: Great Smokies Diagnostic Laboratory, *Interpretive Guidelines for Amino Acid Analysis*

Quick Reference

The following provides at a glance reference for specific conditions. Everybody's needs are unique and some nutrients may work better for you than others. For specifics including amounts, go to the appropriate section in this book.

Anti-Aging
Nutritional support includes methionine, 5-THP, glutamine, Ester C, BNC + GABA, melatonin, pycnogenol (OPC), huperzine A, antioxidants.
Avoid chemicals and pesticides.

Aggressiveness
Nutritional support includes 5-HTP, GABA, glycine, glutamine, taurine, tyrosine, B6 (timed-release), Liquid Serotonin.
Avoid phenylalanine, sugar.

Alzheimer's Disease
Nutritional support includes BNC + GABA, glutamine, ginkgo, B6 (timed-release), pycnogenol (OPC), Ester C, DMG, phosphatidylserine, Huperzine A (*Do not use if heart or pulmonary disease is present.*), B12 injections, DHEA, Mag Link.
Avoid processed foods, alcohol, cigarette smoke, pesticides, and the minerals, aluminum and mercury.

Arthritis (Osteo)
Nutritional support includes histidine, cysteine, BNC + GABA, boswella, glucosamine, chrondroitin, Malic Acid Plus, DLPA, Ester C, magnesium (Mag Link), MSM, niacinamide, shark cartilage.
Avoid nightshade foods (PPET)—peppers, potatoes, eggplant, and tomatoes, processed foods, dairy products, and red meat.

Autism
Nutritional support includes Brain Link Complex, HTP10, B6 or P5'P, 5-HTP, glutamine, magnesium, Liquid Serotonin.

Body Building
Nutritional support includes BCAA, alanine, carnitine, ornithine, Alpha KG, creatine.

Cancer
Nutritional support includes cysteine, taurine, glutamine, BNC + GABA, Ester C, antioxidants, BCAA, melatonin, pycnogenol (OPC), Brain Link Complex.
Avoid phenylalanine and tyrosine with melanoma, or if you have a history of a melanoma; pesticides, chemical exposure.
For a detailed program on cancer, refer to *Definitive Guide to Cancer* by W. John Diamond, M.D., et al.

Cholesterol
Nutritional support includes carnitine, methionine, arginine, glycine, taurine, chromium picolinate, fortified flax, CoEnzyme Q10.
Avoid saturated fats. Use monounsaturated fats such as olive or canola oils. Be aware many anti-cholesterol drugs lower your CoQ10 levels, putting you at risk.

Chronic Illness
Nutritional support includes BCAA, BNC + GABA, cysteine, glutamine, 5-HTP, Ester C, antioxidants, pycnogenol (OPC). Increase organic foods.
Avoid pesticides and chemicals.

Chronic Pain
Nutritional support includes 5-HTP, DLPA, GABA, glutamine, BNC + GABA, boswella, magnesium (Mag Link), Ester C, PoweRelief, Mobigesic.
Avoid pain medications as you buildup a tolerance and require more drugs to get relief. Many pain medications are addictive.

Cirrhosis/GI Healing
Nutrients support includes glutamine, carnitine, BCAA, CoQ10.

Depression
Nutritional support includes 5-HTP, phenylalanine, tyrosine, methionine, GABA, carnitine, threonine, taurine, Mood Sync, St. John's Wort, and Mag Link.
Avoid arginine. Use *extreme* caution if combining with antidepressant medications. See specifics in this book or talk with a pharmacist.

Diabetes
Nutritional support includes 5-HTP, carnitine, taurine, chromium picolinate, Mag Link (magnesium chloride tabs), pycnogenol, Ester C, Vitamin E, vanadium, alpha lipoic acid.
Avoid simple sugars.

Drug Addiction
Nutritional support includes GABA, tyrosine, glutamine, methionine, DLPA, B-complex, 5-HTP, B6 (timed-release), Mood Sync, Anxiety Control.
Avoid alcohol and drugs.

Energy
Nutritional support includes carnitine, tyrosine or phenylalanine, CoQ10, Alpha KG. If over 40, consider supplementing with DHEA 25 to 50 mg.
Avoid food (sensitivities or allergies) that causes fatigue.

Epilepsy
Nutritional support includes glycine, GABA, taurine, B6, melatonin, 5-HTP.
Avoid strobe lights, pesticides, and chemicals.

Gallbladder
Nutritional support includes taurine, methionine, glycine, BCAA, digestive enzymes, pancreatin, ginger.
Avoid fatty foods.

Heart Failure
Nutritional support includes taurine, tyrosine, carnitine, BCAA, CoEnzyme Q10, Mag Link (magnesium chloride tabs).

Herpes/Shingles (Herpes Zoster)
Nutritional support includes lysine, Ester C, Vitamin B-complex, VitaminE, Vitamin B12 injectable, PoweRelief, DLPA.
Avoid arginine.

Hyperactivity
Nutritional support includes GABA, glycine, glutamine, taurine, Brain Link Complex, 5-HTP, Liquid Serotonin, BNC + GABA, HTP10, Mood Sync or Teen Link.

Hypertension
Nutritional support includes 5-HTP, GABA, taurine, Mag Link (magnesium chloride tabs), calcium, CoEnzyme Q10, Anxiety Control or Mood Sync.
Avoid stimulants, anger, and emotional upsets.

Hypoglycemia
Nutritional support includes alanine, GABA, chromium picolinate, vanadium, Mag Link (magnesium chloride tabs), gymnema sylvestre, alpha lipoic acid.

Insomnia
Nutritional support includes 5-HTP, melatonin, GABA, Mood Sync, Mag Link (magnesium chloride tabs).
Avoid phenylalanine.

Leg Ulcers
Nutritional support includes topical cysteine, glycine, threonine, BCAA, Ester C, zinc, Mag Link (magnesium chloride).

Liver Disease
Nutritional support includes BCAA, carnitine, glutamine, B6.

Mania
Nutritional support includes 5-HTP, GABA, glycine, BNC + GABA, glutamine.
Avoid phenylalanine, tyrosine, and stimulants.

Memory/Concentration
Nutritional support includes glutamine, GABA, ginkgo, Huperzine A, Acetyl-L-Carnitine, BNC + GABA, B6 (timed-release).

Mental Alertness
Nutritional support includes tyrosine, phenylalanine, glutamine, ginkgo.

Parkinson's Disease
Nutritional support includes phenylalanine, tyrosine, 5-HTP, methionine, Mag Link (magnesium chloride), Ester C.

Radiation
Nutritional support includes cysteine, glutamine, taurine, Ester C, beta-carotene, pycnogenol.

Renal Failure
Nutritional support includes BNC + GABA, carnitine, BCAA.

Schizophrenia
Nutritional support includes GABA, isoleucine, 5-HTP, methionine, B6, non-flush niacin.
Avoid serine, leucine, asparagine. Check for food allergies.

Seizures
Nutritional support includes taurine, GABA, Mag Link.

Stress
Nutritional support includes Anxiety Control, tyrosine, GABA, BNC + GABA, glutamine, glycine, histidine, ashwagandha, ginseng, Ester C, Mag Link (magnesium chloride).
Avoid sugar in all forms.

Surgery
Nutritional support includes BCAA, BNC + GABA, glutamine, Ester C, beta-carotene.

Tardive Dyskinesia
Nutritional support includes GABA, taurine, BCAA, glutamine, Mag Link (magnesium chloride).

Tobacco Addiction
Nutritional support includes tyrosine, GABA, 5-HTP, glutamine, methionine, B Complex, Sulfonil.
Avoid trying to stop more than one addiction at a time. Do not try to stop drinking caffeine at the same time you are trying to stop smoking.

Weight Control
Nutritional support includes 5-HTP, phenylalanine, GABA, tyrosine, HCA. (Do not use phenylalanine or tyrosine if you are have PKU, pregnant or lactating, have history of melanoma, or use MAO or tricyclic antidepressants).

Amino Acids and Metabolic Pathways
Detoxifying amino acids include cysteine, glutamine, glycine, methionine, taurine, and tyrosine.
Immuno-stimulating amino acids include alanine, aspartic acid, cysteine, glycine, lysine, and threonine.

Drug-Nutrient Actions

Drug/ Condition	Parallel Nutrient	Opposite Nutrient
Anticonvulsants	Taurine, GABA, Glycine, 5-HTP, Magnesium	Aspartic Acid
Antidepressants	Phenylalanine, Tyrosine, Methionine,Taurine, St. John's Wort	Glycine, Histidine
Heart Failure	Taurine, CoEnzyme Q10, Carnitine, Magnesium	Niacin, 5-HTP
High Cholesterol / Triglycerides	Carnitine, Magnesium, Chromium Picolinate	
Steroids (anabolic)	BCAA, Carnitine	Glutamic Acid
Viral antagonists	Lysine, Zinc	Arginine

Product Information

The *purity* of amino acids and nutritional supplements is very important to your success. Be selective. Your body responds to what you absorb. Absorption enhances when you *use only pharmaceutical-grade products.*

There are four grades of supplemental amino acids and nutritional products. We list them in order of purity from least pure to purest—food lot, cosmetic, pharmaceutical grade, I.V. grade.

Pharmaceutical grade generally guarantees purity of product. Capsules are generally cleaner and purer than tablets, and *more bioavailable.* Tablets require fillers and binders. When considering nutritional supplements, look for preservative-free and excipient-free products because they are better. Buy supplements that are free of preservatives, fillers, binders, or excipients of any kind. *Insist on pharmaceutical-grade products. Your body and brain will know the difference.*

For information on products and other books, call 1-800-669-2256 or visit Pain & Stress Center website: http://www.painstresscenter.com

Bibliography

Aatron Medical Services, Inc. *Amino Acids Metabolism and Analysis.* 1989.

Amaducci L., et al. "Use of phosphatidylserine in Alzheimer's Disease." *Annuals New York Academy of Science.* Vol. 640, 1991, pp. 245–249.

Babal, Ken. "The Fall and Rise of Tryptophan," *Nutrition Science News,* February, 1998, Vol. 3, No. 2, pp. 60–64.

Balch, James F. and Phyllis A. Balch. *Prescription for Nutritional Healing.* Garden City Park, NY: Avery Publishing Group, 1997.

Barbeau, A. *Archives of Neurology.* Vol. 30, 1982, pp. 52–58.

Barbeau, Andre and Ryan J. Huxtable. *Taurine.* New York, NY: Raven Press, 1975.

Barbeau, Andre and Ryan J. Huxtable. *Taurine and Neurological Disorders.* New York, NY: Raven Press, 1978.

Birdsall, Timothy C. "Therapeutic Applications of Taurine." *Alternative Medicine Review.* Vol. 3, No. 2, 1998, pp. 128–136.

Bland, Jeffrey, Ed. *Medical Applications of Clinical Nutrition.* New Canaan, CT: Keats Publishing, 1983.

Bland, Jeffrey S. Psychoneuro-Nutritional Medicine: An Advancing Paradigm. *Alternative Therapies.* May, 1995, pp. 22–27.

Block, K.O. and M. Friedman. *Absorption and Utilization of Amino Acids.* Boca Raton: CRC Press, Volume 1, 1989.

Bliznakov, and Gerald L. Hunt. *The Miracle Nutrient: CoEnzyme Q10.* New York: Bantam Books, 1987, pp. 65–123.

Bowery, N.G., et al. (ed.) *GABA$_B$ Receptors in Mammalian Function.* New York: John Wiley & Sons, 1990.

Brain Research Bulletin. Vol. 48, pp. 203–209.

Bralley, J. Alexander and Richard S. Lord, Eds. *Laboratory Evaluations in Nutritional Medicine.* June/October 1999, pp. 4–19.

Breggin, Peter. *Talking Back to Ritalin.* Monroe, ME: Common Courage Press, 1998.

Breggin, Peter. *Toxic Psychiatry.* New York: St. Martin's Press, 1991.

Braverman, Eric and Carl C. Pfeiffer. *The Healing Nutrients Within.* New Canaan, CT: Keats Publishing, Inc., 1987.

Carter, Rita. *Mapping the Mind.* Berkeley, CA: University of California Press, 1998, p. 23.

Cenacchi T. et al. "Cognitive decline in the elderly: A double-bind, placebo-controlled multicenter study on efficacy of phosphatidylserine administration." *Aging Clinical Experimental Research.* Vol. 5. 1993, pp. 123–133.

Chaitow, Leon. *Thorsons Guide to Amino Acids.* London: Thorsons, 1991.

Chen, L.H. "Biomedical Influences on Nutrition of the Elderly." *Nutritional Aspects of Aging.* Boca Raton: CRC Press, 1986.

Cooper, Jack R., et al. *The Biochemical Basis of Neuropharmacology* New York: Oxford University Press, 1990.

Crook, T.H., et al. "Effects of Phosphatidylserine in Age-Associated Memory Impairment." *Neurology,* Vol. 41, 1991, pp. 644–649.

Crook, T, et al. "Effects of phosphatidylserine in Alzheimer's disease." *Psychopharmacolgy Bulletin.* Vol. 28, 1992, pp. 61–66.

Cross, L.D. "Carpal Tunnel Syndrome, Epidemic of the 90s." *Health Naturally.* April/May, 1998, pp. 34–37.

Davies, Stephen and Alan Stewart. *Nutritional Medicine (Vol 1).* New York: Avon Books, 1987.

Davis, Joel. *Endorphins, New Wave of Brain Chemistry.* New York, NY: The Dial Press, 1984.

Devlin, T. M. *Textbook of Biochemistry.* New York, NY: Wiley, 1982.

Dodson W., Sach D., Krauss S., et al. "Alterations of serum and urinary carnitine profiles in cancer patients. Hypothesis of possible significance. *Journal Ameican College of Nutrition.* Vol. 8, 1989, pp. 133–142.

Ellis, John M. and Jean Pamplin. Vitamin B6 Therapy. Garden City Park: Avery Publishing, 199, pp. 1–45, 101–150.

Formica, P.E. "The housewife syndrome: treatment with the potassium and magnesium salts of aspartic acid." *Current Therapy Research.* Vol. 4, 1962, p. 98.

"Four Prespectives on Carpal Tunnel Syndrome," *Your Health.* Asheville, NC: International Academy of Nutrition and Preventive Medicine. Vol. XIII No. III, 1992.

Fox, Arnold and Barry Fox. *DLPA To End Chronic Pain and Depression.* New York: Long Shadow Books, 1985.

Gaby, Alan. *B6, The Natural Healer.* New Canaan, CT: Keats Publishing, 1984.

Gaby, Alan R. *Magnesium.* New Canaan, CT: Keats Publishing, 1994.

Gaster, Barak. "S-adenosylmethionine (SAMe) for the Treatment of Depression." *Alternative Medicine Alert.* December 1999, p. 133–135.

Gelenberg, A. J. et al. "Tyrosine treatment of depression." *American Journal of Psychiatry.* Vol. 137, 1980, p. 622.

Gerber, James. *Handbook of Therapeutic and Preventative Nutrition.* Gaithersburg, MD: Aspen, 1993, pp. 244–245.

Gitlin, Michael. *The Psychotherapist's Guide to Psychopharmacology.* New York: The Free Press, 1990.

Goldberg, Burton, et al. *Alternative Medicine Guide to Heart Disease.* Tiburon, CA: Future Medicine Publishing. 1998.

Granat, Q. and J. DiMichele. "Phosphatidylserine in Elderly Patients. An Open Trial." *Clinical Trials Journal.* Vol. 24, 1987, pp. 99–103.

Griffith, R, D.Delong, and C. Kagan. Dermatologia. No. 156, pp. 257–267, 1978.

Harrison, Tinsley R., Thorn, George W. (ed), et al. *Harrison's Principles of Internal Medicine.* 8th Ed. New York: McGraw-Hill Book Co, 1977.

Hicks, J.T. "Treatment of fatigue in general practice: a double-blind study." *Clinical Medicine.* January 1964, p. 85.

Hoffer, Abram and Morton Walker. *Orthomolecular Nutrition.* New Canaan, CT: Keats Publishing, 1978.

Hosking G.P., N.P. Cavanaugh, D.P. Symth, et al. "Oral treatment of Carnitine Mypopathy." *Lancet.* Vol. 16, 1977, p. 853.

Huxtable, R. J. and H. Pasantes-Morales. *Taurine in Nutrition and Neurology.* New York, NY: Plenium Press, 1981.

Huxtable, R. J. "Physiological Actions of Taurine." *Physiology Review.* Vol. 72, pp. 101–103.

Harper, H. A. *Review of Physiological Chemistry.* 12th Ed. Los Altos, CA: Lange Medical Publications, 1969, p. 29.

Isaacs H., J. Heffron, M. Badenhorst, et al. "Weakness Associated with the Pathological Presence of Lipid in Skeletal Muscle: A Detailed Study of a Patient with Carnitine Deficiency." *Journal of Neurology, Neurosurgery and Psychiatry.* Vol. 39, 1976, pp. 1114–1123.

"Is Dietary Cholesterol Really Public Enemy #1?" *Women's Health Connection.* Vol. VI, Issue I.

Kagan, C. "Lysine Therapy for Herpes Simplex." *The Lancet.* Vol. 1, No. 37, 1974.

Kaltz, Ronald and Carol Kahn. *Grow Young with HGH.* New York: Harper Collins, 1998.

Kotulak, Ronald. *Inside the Brain.* Kansas City: Andrew and McMeel, 1996.

Kruse, C.A. "Treatment of fatigue with aspartic acid salts." *Northwest Medicine.* June 1961, p. 257.

Lacour, B., S. DiGiulio, J. Chanard, et al. "Carnitine improves lipid anomalies in hemodialysis patient." *Lancet.* October 11, 1978, pp. 763–764.

Lee, John R. with Virginia Hopkins. *What Your Doctor May Not Tell You About Menopause.* New York: Warner Books, 1996, pp. 64, 285, 300–305.

Leibovitz, Brian. *Carnitine, The Bt Phenomenon. 1984.*

Lemon, P.W.R. and J.P. *Journal of Applied Physiology.* 1980, pp. 624–629.

Li, J.B., Jefferson, L.S. *Biochemical Biophysical Acta.* 1978, pp. 351–359.

Maher, Timothy J. "L-Arginine Continuing Education Module." New Hope Institute. February 2000, pp. 2–7.

Mervyn, Len. *Minerals and Your Health.* New Canaan, CT: Keats Publishing, 1980, pp.36–40, 79–81.

Milne, Robert, et. al. *Definitive Guide to Headaches.* Tiburon, CA: Future Medicine Publishing, 1998.

Moore, Thomas. *Prescription for Disaster.* New York: Simon & Schuster, 1998.

Mowrey, Daniel. *Herbal Tonic Therapies.* New Canaan, CT: Keats Publishing, 1993

Moyers, Bill. *Healing and the Mind.* New York: Doubleday, 1993.

Murray, Michael T. *The Healing Power of Herbs.* Rocklin, CA: Prima Publishing, 1995, p. 208.

Murray, Michael T. "The Many Benefits of Carnitine." *The American Journal of Natural Medicine.* March, 1966., pp. 6–13.

Newbold, H.L. *Mega-Nutrients for Your Nerves.* New York: Peter Wyden, Publishing, 1975.

Neuborne, Ellen. "Workers in pain; employers up in arms." *USA Today,* January 9, 1997, Section B, p. 1–2.

Pasantes-Morales, Herminia et al. eds. *Taurine: Functional Neurochemistry, Physiology, and Cardiology.* New York: Wiley-Liss, 1990.

Pert, Candace B. *Molecules of Emotion.* New York: Scribner Publishing, 1997.

Pfeiffer, Carl. Mental and Elemental Nutrition. New Canaan, CT: Keats Publishing, 1975.

Pfeiffer, Carl. *Nutrition and Mental Illness.* Rochester, VT: Healing Arts Press, 1987.

Poortmans, J.R., and In. H. Howard H. *Metabolic Adaptation to Prolonged Physical Exercise.* Bsel, Switzerland: Birkhauseer Verlag, 1975, p. 212–228.

Prusinev, Stanley. *The Enzymes of Glutamine Metabolism.* New York, NY: Academic Press, 1973.

Rapp, Doris. *Is This Your Child's World?* New York: Bantam Books, 1996.

Rogers, L.L. "Glutamine in the Treatment of Alcoholism." *Quarterly Journal of Studies on Alcohol.* Vol. 18, No. 4., 1957, pp. 581–587.

Rogers, L.L. and R.B. Pelton. "Effect of Glutamine on IQ Scores of Mentally Deficient Children." *Texas Reports on Biology and Medicine.* Vol. 15, No. 1, 1957, pp. 84–90.

Sahley, Billie J. *The Anxiety Epidemic.* San Antonio, Texas: Pain & Stress Publications, 1999.

Sahley, Billie J. and Katherine M. Birkner. *Breaking Your Prescribed Addiction.* San Antonio, TX: Pain & Stress Publications, 1998.

Sahley, Billie J. *Control Hyperactivity and A.D.D./A.D.H.D. Naturally.* San Antonio, TX: Pain & Stress Publications®, 2000.

Sahley, Billie J. *GABA, The Anxiety Amino Acid.* San Antonio, TX: Pain & Stress Publications®, 1998.

Shabert, Judy and Nancy Ehrlich. *The Ultimate Nutrient, Glutamine.* Garden City Park, NY: Avery Publishing, 1994.

Shaw, D.L. et al. "Management of fatigue: a physiological approach." *American Journal Medical Science.* 1962, pp. 243, 758.

Smith, Robert. "Chronic Headaches in Family Practice." *Journal of the American Board of Family Practice.* Vol. 6, Nov/Dec, 1992, pp. 589–599.

Souba, Wiley W., et al. "Glutamine Metabolism by the Intestinal Tract." *Journal of Parenteral and Enteral Nutrition.* Vol. 9., No. 5 p. 608.

Thompsen J.H., A.L. Shug, V.U. Yap, et al: "Improved pacing tolerance of the ischemic human myocardium after administration of carnitine." *American Journal of Cardiology.* Vol. 43, 1979, pp. 300–305.

Thomson, J. et al. "The treatment of depression in general practice: a comparison of L-tryptophan, amitriptyline and combination with placebo." *Psychological Medicine.* December 1982, p. 741

Tischler, M. et al. *Journal Biological Chemistry.* Vol. 4, pp. 1613–1621.

"Riboflavin Zaps Migraines." *Vitamin Retailer.* May, 1998, pp. 53–54.

Werbach, Melvyn. *Nutritional Influences on Illness.* Tarzana, CA: Third Line Press, 1987, pp. 73, 119, 138–139, 192–193, 200.

Whitaker, Julian. "Diabetes Treatment Review: How to Take Control," *Health and Healing Newsletter.* September, 1995, pp. 1–4.

Whitaker, Julian. *Reversing Diabetes.* New York: Warner Books, 1987.

White, A. et al. *Principles of Biochemistry.* 6th Ed. New York, NY: McGraw-Hill, 1978.

Williams, R.J. *Alcoholism: The Nutritional Approach.* Austin, TX: Univ. of Texas Press, 1958, pp. 88, 100.

Wilson, Eva D. et al. *Principles of Nutrition.* New York: John Wiley & Sons, 1979, pp. 274–275.

"Women and Sex Drive." *Life Enhancement,* December 1999, pp. 4–8.

Zheng, J.J. and I.H. Rosenberg. "What is the Nutritional Status of the Elderly?" *Geriatrics.* June, 1989, pp. 57–64.

Index

About the Authors

Billie J. Sahley, Ph.D., is Executive Director of the Pain & Stress Center in San Antonio. She is a Board Certified Medical Psychotherapist-Behavior Therapist, and an Orthomolecular Therapist. She is a Diplomate in the American Academy of Pain Management. Dr. Sahley is a graduate of the University of Texas, Clayton University School of Behavioral Medicine, and U.C.L.A. School of Integral Medicine. Additionally, she has studied advanced nutritional biochemistry through Jeffrey Bland, Ph.D., Director of HealthComm. She is a member of the Huxley Foundation/Academy of Orthomolecular Medicine, Academy of Psychosomatic Medicine, North American Nutrition and Preventive Medicine Association. In addition, she holds memberships in the American Academy of Environmental Medicine, Sports Medicine Foundation, and American Mental Health Counselors Association. She also sits on the Scientific and Medical Advisory Board for Inter-Cal Corporation.

Dr. Sahley wrote: *The Anxiety Epidemic; Control Hyperactivity/A.D.D. Naturally; Chronic Emotional Fatigue; Malic Acid and Magnesium For Fibromyalgia and Chronic Pain Syndrome; The Melatonin Report; Is Ritalin Necessary? The Ritalin Report;* and has recorded numerous audio cassette tapes. She coauthored *Breaking Your Prescribed Addiction.*

In addition, Dr. Sahley holds three U.S. patents for: SAF, Calms Kids (SAF For Kids), and Anxiety Control 24.

Kathy Birkner is a Pain Therapist at the Pain & Stress Center in San Antonio. She is a Registered Nurse, Certified Registered Nurse Anesthetist, and Orthomolecular Therapist. She is a Diplomate in the American Academy of Pain Management. She attended Brackenridge Hospital School of Nursing, University of Texas at Austin, Southwest Missouri State University, and Clayton University. She holds degrees in nursing, nutrition, and behavior therapy. Dr. Birkner has done graduate studies through the Center for Integral Medicine and U.C.L.A. Medical School under the direction of Dr. David Bresler. Additionally, she has studied advanced nutritional biochemistry through Jeffrey Bland, Ph.D., Director of HealthComm. She is a member of American Association of Nurse Anesthetists, Texas Association of Nurse Anesthetists, American Association of Pain Management, American College of Osteopathic Pain Management and Sclerotherapy, American Holistic Nurse Association, and American Association of Counseling and Development. She is author of *Breaking Your Sugar Habit Cookbook* and coauthor with Dr. Sahley of the audio cassette tape, *Therapeutic Uses of Amino Acids,* and *Breaking Your Prescribed Addiction* book.